12

MINISTRY OF
AGRICULTURE, FISHERIES AND FOOD

MANUAL OF NUTRITION

LONDON
HER MAJESTY'S STATIONERY OFFICE
1970

First published 1945
Seventh Edition 1970
Third impression 1975

ISBN 0 11 240965 2

Contents

Introduction . . . . *Page* 1

PART I

Carbohydrates 5
Fats 7
Proteins 9
Food Consumption and Physical Work . . 12

PART II

Inorganic Elements 19
Vitamins 24

PART III

Digestion of Foods and Absorption of Nutrients . 34
Recommended Nutrient Intakes 40
Composition of Food 45

PART IV

Cooking 53
Meals 61
Planning Balanced Meals 65
Methods of Teaching Nutrition 71

APPENDICES

A. Composition of Food 75
B. Scheme for Lectures 100
C. Suggested Demonstrations 101
D. Recommended Books 102

DIAGRAM

The Digestive System 34

Foreword

THIS booklet is designed to provide the reader with a working knowledge of nutrition and the principles upon which it is based. First published in 1945, the Manual of Nutrition was originally the work of Dr. Magnus Pyke who was at that time a member of the Scientific Adviser's Division of the Ministry of Food. The present edition, the seventh, has been prepared by members of the Food Science Advice Branch of the Ministry of Agriculture, Fisheries and Food in consultation with other Departments and the text and tables have been thoroughly revised. The metric system of units has been used to calculate the amounts of different nutrients in food, but some of the traditional units are also retained and the inter-relationship is shown.

Before even a broad assessment of the nutritional value of individual foods or of diets can be made it is necessary to know something of the chemical composition of the commoner foods and the effects on the body of the substances they contain. This information is given in Parts I and II of the Manual and in the tables of food composition in Appendix A. More detailed information on the nutrient content and energy (calorie) value of foods will be found in *The Composition of Foods* by R. A. McCance and E. M. Widdowson (1967)* on which Appendix A is based.

The utilization of foods and their fate in the body is discussed in Part III and this is followed by a section on recommended intakes of nutrients for healthy persons living in the United Kingdom. The figures given in the Table on page 42 are those recommended by the Department of Health and Social Security in a report published in 1969. To be satisfactory, any diet or daily menu pattern must contain adequate amounts of all the nutrients and these recommendations may be used as guides in menu planning. The effects of storage, food processing and cooking on the ultimate nutrient content of food served on the plate are considered briefly in Part IV. From this introduction it can be seen that the science of nutrition forms part of a complex of subjects which demands careful study; moreover, no attempt has been made in this short booklet to teach chemistry, physiology or any other basic subject upon which nutrition is founded. Those who master the material set out in the following pages cannot claim to be specialists in nutrition or dietetics but it is hoped that the knowledge gained will provide a starting point for those who may be stimulated to make a more detailed study of the different facets of nutrition; to assist them a comprehensive list of books for further reading has been included.

Ministry of Agriculture, Fisheries and Food

September 1970

---

* Medical Research Council Special Report Series No 297 HMSO

Introduction

THE foods eaten by the peoples of the world may vary widely among different countries and even among the districts within them, but any diet must contain sufficient foods of chemically different kinds if the health of the individual is not to suffer. The science of nutrition includes the study of those principles by which the sufficiency of a diet can be measured. Anyone whose business it is to provide meals should know the fundamentals of nutrition and be able thereby to estimate the value of the food provided.

It is necessary, first, to define certain terms in common use.

The science of NUTRITION is the study of all processes of growth, maintenance and repair of the living body that depend upon the intake of food.

LIFE, here considered as the state of continual change and functional activity which distinguishes animals and vegetables from inanimate matter, is, from a nutritional point of view, a chemical process by which an organism draws from food the material and energy necessary for its growth, continuity of existence and power of reproduction.

FOOD is, for the purposes of this booklet, any solid or liquid which, when swallowed, can do one or more of three things:

(*a*) furnish the body with material from which it can produce heat, work, or other forms of energy;

(*b*) provide material to enable growth, repair or reproduction to proceed;

(*c*) supply substances which participate in the mechanisms regulating the production of energy or the processes of growth, repair and reproduction. The foods in this group are sometimes known as the protective foods because they help to maintain health.

The diet may be chosen from a very large number of foods, all of which contain one or more of the groups of materials listed below. These components, which give a substance its right to be called a food, are known as 'nutrients'. A balanced diet is one which contains all the nutrients in the required proportions. (See also pages 44 and 65).

NUTRIENTS IN FOODS

Carbohydrates provide the body with energy and may also be converted into body fat.

Fats provide energy and may also form body fat.

Proteins provide materials for growth and repair of body tissues. They can also provide energy and sometimes can be converted into fat.

Mineral substances provide material for growth and repair, and for regulation of body processes.

Vitamins regulate the body processes

Water and oxygen from the air are necessary for life, but are not here classified as nutrients.

A nutrient may be said to be 'essential' when it cannot be synthesized by the body, at least in sufficient quantity.

Very few foods contain only one nutrient; most are mixtures and contain several. The importance of a particular food in terms of nutrients depends as much on the quantity in which it is eaten as on the amount of a nutrient present in a given quantity. Thus, parsley which is rich in vitamin C is not as valuable as potatoes which, although containing less vitamin C on a weight for weight basis, are eaten in considerably larger amounts.

The need of the body for water is second only to its need for air. Approximately two-thirds of the body weight consists of water; water transports food to the body cells and carries away the waste products. The body is continually balancing the amount of water taken in the diet with the amount excreted. If too much is drunk the excess is excreted through the kidneys; if too little, dehydration occurs. In a temperate climate at least one litre ($1\frac{3}{4}$ pt) of water or other fluid should be drunk daily; more is needed if physical work is done or the weather is hot.

MALNUTRITION

The maintenance of nutrition in an individual depends on the provision of appropriate quantities of all the nutrients; too little or too much of some may lead to a condition of *malnutrition*. An insufficient total quantity of nutrients results in *under-nutrition* of which the extreme degree is *starvation*. (See page 18).

The stunting of a child's physical or mental development from lack of protein or other nutrients, or the cracking and ulceration of an adult's lips from shortage of vitamins, may be described as resulting from malnutrition as may excessive fatness from the consumption of too much food. Obesity is associated with much ill health and in severe degrees with a greatly increased mortality rate.

CHEMICAL PROCESS OF LIVING

The body derives from food its energy and its material for growth and self-maintenance. Wheat can be treated in a laboratory to produce measurable heat, that is, energy, and this property has been exploited in times of glut when the grain has been used for fuel in railway engines. Whether wheat is used in engines or as a food by the body an almost identical amount of energy is produced. The chemical apparatus of the body differs, of course, from that of the laboratory or engine, but the overall result is the same. Again, the process by which petrol enables the wheels of a car to turn is chemical; so is the process by which food empowers a muscle to move a limb. The characteristic difference between the processes is that the apparatus of the body ensures that the release of energy takes place only gradually in a long series of controlled, discrete steps. Each step is mediated by an enzyme.

Enzymes

Enzymes are substances which must be present for the reactions involved in the metabolism of food to proceed correctly. They are catalysts in that they influence the rate of reactions, but do not form any part of the resultant products. Chemically enzymes are complex protein compounds, which are synthesized by the body. They may be classified according to the type of reaction they control and are generally highly specific to one particular substance concerned in the reactions. Some enzymes will not function by themselves and require the presence of a *cofactor* to activate them. Many vitamins and minerals are concerned in these enzyme systems; they cannot be synthesized by the human body and must therefore be supplied in the diet as such.

MULTIPLE FUNCTION OF FOOD

From the definition of food given above, it may be said that iron, even in the form of rust from a cooking pot, is a food, since it may be used to renew substances in the blood. Nevertheless this definition of food is imperfect and must be used with discretion. For example, alcohol is a food in that it can provide energy, but it is also a narcotic drug. Small amounts of iodine rank as food, for iodine normally regulates a function of the body; but iodine in excess is a poison. Substances which can regulate body function, but are simply drugs, are excluded by the definition from classification as foods; but the two examples alcohol and iodine—there are many others—illustrate the difficulty of deciding what is a food and what is not. Salt, which helps to repair the body and regulate its functions, is a food; pepper is not.

STANDARD MEASUREMENTS OF AMOUNT

Standard units must be used to calculate the amount of different nutrients in food. The metric system (in the form known as SI*) is being increasingly used in all fields and is used in this edition of the Manual; some of the

Common symbols and conversion factors

Weight	microgram	µg	Ounce	oz
	milligram	mg	pound	lb
	gram	g	stone	st
	kilogram	kg		
	1 g = 1,000 mg		1 g = 0·035 oz	
	= 1,000,000 µg		1 kg = 2·20 lb	
	1 kg = 1,000 g		1 oz = 28·35 g	
			1 lb = 453·6 g	
			1 st = 6·35 kg	
Volume	millilitre	ml	fluid ounce	fl oz
	litre	l	pint	pt
	1 l = 1,000 ml		1 fl oz = 28·4 ml	
			1 pt = 20 fl oz	
			1 pt = 568 ml	
Energy	joule	J	Kilocalorie	kcal
	kilojoule	kJ		
	megajoule	MJ		
	1 kJ = 1,000 J		1 kcal = 4·19 kJ	
	1 MJ = 1,000 kJ		1 MJ = 239 kcal	
	= 1,000,000 J			

International units (i.u.) have been used in the past for a number of vitamins as an agreed measurement of their value to the body, but units of weight are to be preferred.

* The 'Système International d'Unités' in which there are units for six basic physical quantities, which include length and mass, and a number of other units for derived physical quantities such as energy, force and power.

traditional units are also retained. Inter-relations between units are shown above.

The energy value of food is commonly measured in terms of heat units called calories. In nutritional studies the quantitative unit used is the kilocalorie, which is the amount of heat required to raise the temperature of 1 kilogram of water one degree Centigrade. But it is probable that the kilojoule or megajoule will be increasingly used instead of the kilocalorie.

PART I

Carbohydrates

THERE are three major groups of carbohydrates: sugars, starches and cellulose and related materials; the classification depends upon the size of the molecule. All are composed of carbon, hydrogen and oxygen. The chemical structure of carbohydrates is based on a common pattern, but the units are linked together in different numbers and at different parts of the units.

SUGARS

MONOSACCHARIDES or simple sugars

Glucose, one of the simplest of the sugars, may be made from starch or by splitting a more complex sugar such as sucrose. It occurs naturally in the blood of living animals and in fruit and plant juices. It plays an important part in the body.

Liquid glucose is made by hydrolysing maize starch and it consists of a mixture of glucose, maltose and several other complex sugars, glucose being the single sugar present in highest concentration. It is less sweet than glucose and it is used in medical treatment and in confectionery manufacture.

Fructose forms a part of sucrose from which it may be derived and in some circumstances it may be changed into glucose. It is the sweetest sugar known and occurs naturally in plant juices, fruit and honey.

Galactose does not occur in a free state but forms part of other molecules such as lactose.

DISACCHARIDES are composed of two monosaccharides linked together (minus the elements of water).

Sucrose is a chemical combination of glucose and fructose. It occurs naturally in sugar cane and sugar beet, in sweet fruits and in roots such as carrots.

Lactose, less sweet than sucrose, is a combination of glucose and galactose. It occurs in all types of milk, including human milk.

Maltose is a combination of two glucose molecules. It is formed naturally from starch during the germination of grain and also in the production of malt liquors such as beers.

PROPERTIES OF SUGARS

All sugars, whether monosaccharides or disaccharides, are sweet and soluble in water. They are all capable of forming crystals when the water in which they are dissolved becomes supersaturated with them.

Non-sugar sweeteners are compounds which are also sweet but bear no chemical or nutritional relationship to sugar. An example is *saccharin*, which on a weight basis is about 500 times as sweet as sucrose; being of no value to the body it does not rank as a food. For this reason it may be used as a sweetening agent when it is necessary to restrict the amount of carbohydrate in the diet. *Sorbitol*, made from glucose, can also be used as a sugar substitute and, because it is absorbed slowly, it is sometimes used in diabetic foods; however, its energy value is similar to that of glucose.

STARCH

Although plants form sugar by the action of the sun on their green leaves, they store the sugar in their stems, roots or seeds as *starch*. This group of carbohydrates forms the greater part of the food reserve of plants and provides by far the largest proportion of carbohydrate in man's food. For example, more than half the solid material in cereal grains and in potatoes is composed of starch; the small amounts present in unripe fruits change to sugar as the fruit ripens.

PROPERTIES OF STARCH

Starch is composed of large numbers of glucose units linked to form both straight and branched chains (*amylose* and *amylopectin* respectively) which are associated in molecules of different sizes. It is stored in the plant in the form of granules, which are of a characteristic size and shape for each plant and can be recognized microscopically. Starch granules form a suspension in cold water but do not dissolve; they cannot be easily digested and, consequently, such foods as flour and potatoes are not eaten raw. When heated in the presence of moisture the granules swell and eventually gelatinize to form a starch paste.

When starch is subjected to dry heat *dextrin* is formed; this is more soluble than starch itself but less soluble than sugar. Starch in bread is changed to dextrin when the bread is toasted.

Glycogen is similar to starch in composition. It is the only carbohydrate of animal origin and is made by the body from glucose, deposited in the liver as a reserve store of carbohydrate material and in the muscle as a more immediate source of fuel. After a spell of hard muscular activity the glycogen supply may be almost exhausted. The amount of glycogen in most meat is small as it breaks down to glucose on the death of the animal. It is also found in some shell-fish.

CELLULOSE AND RELATED MATERIALS

These constitute much of the stiffer structure of vegetables and cereal foods. Cellulose forms the cell walls which enclose the starch grains. It is even less soluble than starch and is unavailable to the human body as direct food. It is of some value in giving bulk to the diet. Ruminants can, however, make direct use of cellulose as food, as can some insects. Manufacturing processes have been devised for breaking down the cellulose in sawdust and other materials into the glucose of which it is composed.

Pectin is a complex carbohydrate present in apples and other fruit and in such roots as turnips. It has the property of forming a stiff jelly which causes jam to set. It is of no direct value as a food for man.

SOURCES OF CARBOHYDRATE

All carbohydrates absorbed by the body contribute heat or energy or they may be converted into fat. The list below gives the total available carbohydrate in different foods.

Almost all foods contain more than a single nutrient. Among the few exceptions is white sugar, which is 100 per cent carbohydrate. Bread, which ranks highly as a source of carbohydrate, also provides substantial amounts of protein and other nutrients.

*Available carbohydrate content of certain foods**

	g per 100 g	g per oz		g per 100 g	g per oz
Sugar	105†	29·8	White bread	54·6	15·5
Syrup	79·0	22·4	Potatoes	18·0	5·1
White flour	80·0	22·7	Bananas, peeled	19·2	5·5
Oatmeal	72·8	20·6	Beans, baked	17·3	4·9
Jam	69·2	19·6	Milk	4·8	1·4
Sultanas	64·7	18·3			

* Expressed as monosaccharide

† More than 100g because expressed as monosaccharide

Main sources of carbohydrate in the diet are bread, flour and other cereals, sugar and preserves and potatoes.

The consumption of sugar per head in Britain has increased six-fold in the last century and a half, while flour consumption has halved. There is evidence that the different dietary carbohydrates have different metabolic consequences, but there is controversy about the significance of these observations in relation to the incidence of diseases such as diabetes and heart disease. However, there is general agreement that excessive consumption of sugar and sweets is detrimental to the teeth, especially when eaten between meals.

Fats

FATS are compounds of *glycerol* with *fatty acids*. The majority are triglycerides in which one unit of glycerol is combined with three fatty acid units. Like carbohydrate, these consist of carbon, hydrogen and oxygen, though in different proportions.

Fatty acids may be either *saturated* or *unsaturated*. If they are saturated, their chemical composition makes them relatively unreactive. On the other hand, unsaturated fatty acids are much more reactive because they possess one or more double bonds between two carbon atoms. They can be changed under certain laboratory and manufacturing conditions to saturated fatty acids by the addition of hydrogen to their double bonds; this process is known as *hydrogenation* and occurs to some extent in the manufacture of margarine when liquid oils are hardened. Nowadays margarines with large amounts of unsaturated fatty acids can be produced. If oxidation occurs at the double bonds, they become rancid.

Some of the more common saturated fatty acids are:

Butyric acid which gives the distinct flavour to butter.

Palmitic acid and *stearic acid* present in most solid fats such as suet.

The more important unsaturated fatty acids are:

Oleic acid found in olive oil and many other vegetable oils.

Linoleic acid found in large amounts in corn oil, soya bean oil, linseed oil and many other vegetable seed oils.

Linolenic acid found in smaller quantities in linseed oil and some vegetable oils.

Arachidonic acid found in very small quantities in some animal fats.

The last three of these acids can be described as *polyunsaturated* because they contain two or more double bonds. They are also called the *essential fatty acids* because they cannot be synthesized by the body and are required in small quantities for normal health. Even longer chain polyunsaturated fatty acids are found in fish oils.

PROPERTIES OF FATS

Fats are insoluble in water; the property which most readily distinguishes them from other components of food is their solubility in such liquids as petrol, chloroform or ether, which are accordingly sometimes described as fat-solvents. Fat-solvents themselves will usually not mix with water.

The physical qualities of fats differ; certain of them become liquid at lower temperatures than others. This depends largely on their degree of unsaturation. Oils are fats which remain liquid at ordinary atmospheric temperatures; if cooled, they become solid.

The energy value of all common fats is roughly equal, although there is evidence that the individual fatty acids of which fats are composed may have different metabolic functions. Some natural fats contain other nutrients of additional value, such as the fat-soluble vitamins A, D and E.

Mineral oils, such as liquid paraffin, are not available for production of body energy and so are not foods.

SOURCES OF FAT

The substances here defined as fats include table fats, all fatty materials such as meat-fat, and all oils derived from animal or vegetable sources.

Fuel for energy can be stored in plants as starch, and in animals as glycogen, but it can be stored in both plants and animals in a more compact form as fat.

In plants, fats are formed from carbohydrate. When seeds such as cotton seed or sunflower seed ripen, their starch content lessens as their fat content increases. Oil seeds, such as these and palm oil, coconut, groundnut, soya bean and palm kernel oils, are among the chief sources of fat for the manufacture of margarine and cooking fat. Most vegetables and fruits contain only traces of fat; the exceptions are the majority of nuts, and soya products.

The fat content of flour and other cereal products, with the exception of oatmeal, is usually low.

In animals, as in plants, fat may be formed from carbohydrate. If more starchy food is eaten than is necessary for the energy expended, fat is laid down in the body. Pigs can be fattened on food largely composed of carbohydrate. Animals, however, can form fat not only from carbohydrate, they can also deposit in their bodies some of the fat from their food. If a pig is given large quantities of cod liver oil, its own body-fat will soon be tainted.

Fish, such as herrings, mackerel, salmon, sardines, pilchards and eels, are sometimes called *fatty fish*. The proportion of fat in them depends, however, on their sexual development and varies with the time of year. *White fish*, such as cod, whiting, haddock and sole, contain very little fat except in the liver.

Oils and fats, such as cooking and salad oils and dripping, are almost 100 per cent fat. Butter is a mixture of butter-fat (from milk), water, certain other nutrients and, usually, added salt. The values given below for the amount of fat in beef and lamb are broadly representative. Meat may, of course, vary widely in fatness. (See also page 13).

Fat content of certain foods

	g per 100 g	g per oz		g per 100 g	g per oz
Salad or cooking oil	99·9	28·3	Bacon	48·0	13·6
Lard, dripping	99·3	28·2	Lamb	31·0	8·8
Margarine	85·3	24·2	Beef	28·2	8·0
Butter	82·5	23·4	Cheese, Cheddar	34·5	9·8
Peanuts	49·0	13·9	Herring	14·1	4·0
			Eggs	12·3	3·5
			Oatmeal	8·7	2·5
			Salmon, canned	6·0	1·7
			Milk	3·8	1·1

Main sources of fat in the diet are butter, margarine and other fats, meat and dairy produce.

Proteins

PROTEINS are compounds of carbon, hydrogen and oxygen and, unlike carbohydrate and fat, they contain nitrogen and sometimes sulphur and phosphorus. They are essential constituents of all living cells and are, therefore, necessary for the growth and repair of the human body. The structure of the proteins of which the human body is made is not the same as that found in plants or animals but the proteins required for human nutrition are built up from the proteins in food (see page 12).

Dietary proteins are split during digestion into their constituent units, *amino acids*. There are about twenty of these commonly found in foods. A single protein will contain several hundred amino acids linked together in a specific arrangement. The number of permutations that can be achieved in this way is virtually infinite; thus the proteins of, for example, beef, beans and cheese are very different from each other because the arrangements and kinds of amino acids in them differ. The body can convert many amino acids of kinds it does not need into amino acids of kinds that it does. There are, however, eight amino acids necessary for the adult and possibly ten for the growing child which cannot be made by the body and must, therefore, be supplied in the diet. These are called the *essential amino acids* and the eight necessary for adults are:

Isoleucine	Phenylalanine
Leucine	Threonine
Lysine	Tryptophan
Methionine	Valine

The two additional ones necessary for the growing child are:

Arginine	Histidine

Proteins in different foods can be graded on the basis of whether they contain the essential amino acids in satisfactory proportions to meet the needs of the body. Such a grading gives a measure of their *biological value*.

Although animal proteins usually contain all the essential amino acids in suitable proportions for human needs, gelatin (derived from meat, fish, gristle and horns) is completely deficient in at least one, tryptophan. Vegetable proteins may be relatively low in one or more of them. With the exception of gelatin, therefore, proteins of animal origin generally have a greater biological value than those of vegetable origin. Such a distinction, however, is often misleading, because mixtures of different plant proteins can have an excellent nutritional value, and the total protein in the diet rarely, if ever, comes from a single source.

There is no method of storing large quantities of individual amino acids in the body. The amino acids in single foods are either used together with other amino acids to make body proteins or they lose their nitrogen and are directly oxidized to supply energy or are converted into carbohydrate or fat. It follows that, for the most efficient use to be made of amino acids in the diet, a complete assortment of those required should be supplied to the body at the same time. This is achieved in practice by eating a mixed diet at each meal, and provides a physiological basis for such favourites as fish and chips and milk with cereals. The capacity of proteins of different origin to make good one another's deficiencies when they are consumed together is known as their *supplementary value*. If the proteins in the diet are to be efficiently utilized the total energy in the diet must be fully adequate for the energy needs of the body.

PROPERTIES OF PROTEINS

Proteins may be classified by their solubility in various solvents.

Egg albumen (the white of egg) is an example of a protein which is water soluble, and this hardens or coagulates during the process of cooking.

Most proteins do not dissolve in water but many common food proteins are soluble in salt and water mixtures of various strengths.

The action of heat on protein is complex. Excessive exposure to heat reduces the nutritive value of protein probably, in part at least, because of the destruction of some amino acids. Thus lysine is partly destroyed during the baking of bread. Under certain conditions a brown discoloration develops during the storage of processed foods, for example, dehydrated vegetables or evaporated milk; this is due to complex reactions between the amino groups and sugars in the food and is known as the Maillard reaction.

SOURCES OF PROTEIN

Plants can build up carbohydrate, and so obtain energy, from substances present in soil and air; in their leaves and roots they can also form their own protein from inorganic materials. Animals cannot form protein in this way, so ultimately must obtain what they need from plants.

There are thus two sources of protein for human nutrition—animal protein and vegetable protein.

Animal Protein

This is a constituent of meat of all kinds, game, poultry, etc.; fish of all kinds, including shell-fish; milk, including dried and condensed forms; cheese and eggs.

Vegetable Protein

The proportion of protein in the plant cells of both green and root vegetables is small. In root vegetables it varies; potatoes contain more than turnips or carrots. Among seeds the proportion is highest in peas and beans; dried peas and beans contain about as much protein as cheese, but the quantity present is diluted when the dried vegetable is soaked in water. Nuts may be grouped with other seeds, having a protein content similar to that of peas and beans, but since they are eaten dry, they are, weight for weight, a better source of protein.

Cereals form the most important class of seed foods. In a grain of cereal, such as wheat, the most active living cells are in the embryo from which, if the grain is planted, the new plant will develop. The larger proportion of the grain consists, however, of the stored starch upon which the plant depends for life until it has developed leaves; it is this starch which makes the grain important as a food for man. The whole grain contains a useful amount of protein but it is not evenly distributed, the embryo and outer layers (bran) being richer. During milling some of the embryo and the parts associated with it are removed, thus reducing the amount of protein in the final flour. Brown flour, therefore, has less protein than the wheat from which it is made but contains more than white flour.

Protein content of certain foods

Animal foods	g per 100 g	g per oz	*Vegetable foods*	g per 100 g	g per oz
Cheese	25·4	7·2	Peanuts	28·1	8·0
Haddock, fillet	16·0	4·5	Peas, dried, raw	21·5	6·1
Beef	14·8	4·2	White flour	10·0	2·8
Lamb	13·0	3·7	Wholemeal bread	9·6	2·7
Eggs	11·9	3·4	White bread	8·3	2·4
Milk	3·3	0·9	Beans, baked	6·0	1·7
			Peas, green	5·8	1·6

Main sources of protein in the diet are meat, dairy produce, bread, flour and other cereals.

USES OF PROTEIN IN THE BODY

Proteins are used for two main purposes: (1) growth and repair, and (2) production of heat and other forms of energy. They are also needed for the formation of enzymes and certain other substances.

1. *For growth and repair.* The protein structure of the human body differs from that of plants, and although similar to that of animals is not identical with it.

If protein in the diet is from vegetable sources, a variety of foods must be eaten in quite large amounts so that the body may have the amounts of different amino acids which it needs to rebuild human tissue. If protein in the diet is from animal sources, less will be needed because it is more like human protein than that from vegetable sources. If protein in the diet is supplied from both animal and vegetable foods, or from a very carefully chosen selection of vegetable foods, the amount required may be as little as if it came from animal sources alone because the variety of amino acids available may enable the body to turn it economically into human protein.

As protein is necessary for growth it follows that growing children and pregnant or nursing women need a greater proportion of protein in their food than adults, who need it for repair and maintenance only. But a certain amount of protein is needed by everybody.

2. *As a source of energy.* In normal circumstances the amount and type of protein in food will not exactly balance requirements for growth and repair; there is usually a proportion of protein material to spare. This is used for production of heat and other energy. Protein has approximately the same energy value as carbohydrate but its fundamental importance in the diet is for growth and repair for which no other nutrient can be a substitute.

Food Consumption and Physical Work

It has been explained that one of the principal uses of food is to supply energy to the living body, and that each of the three nutrients, carbohydrate, fat and protein, of which the diet is composed, can provide this energy. Most foods contain a mixture of these three nutrients; the total energy value of such food is therefore the sum of the energy derived from their carbohydrate, fat and protein. Alcohol can also supply energy.

ENERGY VALUE OF NUTRIENTS

Taking into consideration the composition of different foods and their degrees of absorption by the body it is accepted that:

1 g dietary carbohydrate (as glucose) produces in the body 3·75 kcal or about 16 kJ.
1 g dietary fat produces in the body 9 kcal or about 38 kJ.
1 g dietary protein produces in the body 4 kcal or about 17kJ.
1 g alcohol produces in the body 7 kcal or about 29 kJ.

By using these values the energy content of any food can be calculated from the proportion of nutrients which it contains. For example, white bread contains 15·5 g carbohydrate, 0·5 g fat and 2·4 g protein per oz. The energy value of 1 oz of white bread can be calculated thus:

$$15{\cdot}5 \times 3{\cdot}75 = 58{\cdot}1 \text{ kcal from carbohydrate}$$
$$0{\cdot}5 \times 9 = 4{\cdot}5 \text{ kcal from fat}$$
$$2{\cdot}4 \times 4 = 9{\cdot}6 \text{ kcal from protein}$$

Total 72·2 kcal

However, it is misleading to imply that energy values can be obtained with such precision: decimal points should never be used in the answer, which in this example might be given as 72 or even as 70 kcal. Nevertheless, when doing further calculations, such as the proportion of the energy value derived from protein (13·3 per cent in the example), it is wisest to use the detailed figures, and 'round off' only at the end (i.e., 13 per cent).

ENERGY VALUE OF FOODS

As the energy value of foods is derived from the amounts of nutrients which they contain, it follows that very watery foods (e.g., turnips, lettuce, clear soup) have little energy value. Foods rich in fat have the highest energy value, as shown here:

Energy value of certain foods

	kJ per 100 g	kcal per 100 g	kcal per oz
Cooking fat or lard	3,746	894	253
Butter	3,122	745	211
Bacon	1,994	476	135
Cheese	1,726	412	117
Sugar	1,651	394	112
White flour	1,458	348	99
Beef	1,311	313	89
White bread	1,060	253	72
Dates	1,039	248	70
Herring	796	190	54
Potatoes	318	76	22
Bananas, peeled	318	76	22
Fish, white, fillet	289	69	19
Milk	272	65	18
Apples	193	46	13
Oranges, peeled	147	35	10
Beer, draught mild	105	25	7
Lettuce	46	11	3

Main sources of energy in the diet are bread, flour and other cereals, meat, fats, dairy produce and sugar.

The energy value of meat depends largely on the amount of fat it contains. Meat is mostly composed of the two nutrients, protein and fat, plus water. An increase in the proportion of fat in meat is associated with a decrease in the proportion of water, not of protein; thus the extra fat represents a clear gain to the energy value of the diet. Amounts of fat in two pieces of beef, for example, may of course vary widely; this variation consequently affects the energy value. The composition of other foods may fluctuate similarly; the values given above must therefore be taken as representative only and applied with judgment.

USES OF ENERGY BY THE BODY

Energy from food is used by the body for three purposes:

1. To maintain the processes of living, such as heartbeat and the circulation of blood, breathing and maintenance of body temperature. The energy needed for these processes, when the subject is at complete rest and no physical work is being done, is called the *basal or resting metabolism.*

2. For everyday activities, e.g., standing, eating, moving about and dressing.

3. For performance of *muscular* work (virtually no energy from food is required for mental work).

The amount of energy used by different people for each of the above three purposes depends on the total amount of their living tissues. For many activities energy expenditure is fairly closely related to body weight. Since men are usually larger and heavier than women, their energy needs are greater than those of women. As children are smaller than adults, their need for energy in food is less; on the other hand, children are growing and are more active, so that, although their total needs remain smaller, their needs in proportion to their size are greater than those of adults. Average values for the energy requirements of different categories of people are given in Table 1 on page 42.

ENERGY NEEDED TO MAINTAIN THE PROCESSES OF LIVING

The amount of energy used only for the processes of keeping alive varies from person to person. Representative values for resting metabolism for people in the United Kingdom are as follows:

an adult man weighing 65 kg would require about 1600 kcal per day;
a woman weighing 55 kg would need 1300 kcal;
a child of 8 years of age, weighing 25 kg, would require 1000 kcal;
and a one year old baby (10 kg) about 500 kcal per day.

It is important to appreciate that these are average values. Individuals of these types may need much more, or may survive on much less, but for groups of people these values are representative. During sleep the body needs only its resting requirements, so that if a man sleeps for 8 hours he will use during this period about 500 kcal; a woman would need about 400 kcal. The values expressed in kilojoules or megajoules can be calculated using the factors given on page 3.

FACTORS AFFECTING ENERGY REQUIREMENTS

Body size. Although the energy cost of a particular task to an individual is largely determined by his body weight, surveys have shown that total daily energy expenditure is not closely related to body weight. Big people on average may be less physically active than small people. The figures given in the table on page 42 may be used for calculating the energy needs of groups of people without correlation for body weight.

Age. The basal metabolic rate is high in actively growing young children and falls rapidly in the first 12 years of life. Thereafter it falls more slowly, and after the early twenties it decreases very gradually, largely due to a reduction in the proportion of metabolically active tissue in the body. Also, as people become older they tend to be less physically active and this reduces their energy requirements and thus their need for food.

Physical activity. The degree of activity is the most important variable determining energy requirements, but also the most difficult to assess. Practical ways to deal with this problem are discussed below.

Individual differences in energy requirement. Some people expend more energy and therefore require more from their food than others for performance of a similar day's activity. The estimates given in this chapter apply only to averages, because some individuals get fat on a diet which leaves others thin. The energy need of a particular individual is simply that amount which will enable him to maintain his normal level of activity without—if he is an adult—changing his body weight. This can be found by trial and error.

Climate. The effect of climate on energy requirements need not be considered in the United Kingdom. However, considering the world as a whole, the second Food and Agriculture Organization Committee on Calorie Requirements has recommended that the reference energy requirements should be decreased by 5 per cent for every 10°C (18°F) rise in mean annual temperature *above* the mean reference temperature of 10°C (50°F). But because man is generally more able to protect himself against cold than against heat, the Committee recommended an increase of only 3 per cent for every 10°C (18°F) fall *below* the reference temperature.

ENERGY NEEDED FOR EVERYDAY ACTIVITY OF LIFE

Man's expenditure of just over 1 kcal per minute merely keeps him alive. He needs additional energy every time he moves. However, it is not useful in practice to consider what the additional amount may be, and the following values relate to the *total* energy expended, and therefore required, for different kinds of activity. The values are approximate and appropriate for a normal man; they are given in kcal per minute.

Activity	kcal/min	Activity	kcal/min
Sitting	1·4	Walking slowly	3
Standing	1·7	Walking moderately fast	5
Washing, dressing, etc.	3·5	Walking up and down stairs (overall figure)	9

Everybody, regardless of occupation, needs food to maintain the process of living and for the everyday activity of life; but the decisive factor in the amount of food needed by an individual is the muscular activity of his work and recreation. Examples are given below of a number of physical activities, grouped according to the energy expenditure that they normally entail.

ENERGY NEEDED FOR WORK

Light work
2·5–4·9 kcal/minute
Assembly work
Carpentry
Bricklaying
Most domestic work
Golf

Heavy work
7·5–9·9 kcal/minute
Coal mining
Football
Country dancing

Moderate work
5·0–7·4 kcal/minute
Digging and shovelling
Agricultural work (non-mechanized)
Tennis
Ballroom dancing

Very heavy work
Over 10 kcal/minute
Lumber work
Furnace men (steel industry)
Swimming (crawl)
Cross-country running.

OCCUPATION

Within the same nominal occupation there is wide variation in the nature of the work which is done. Heavy work may only be performed for short periods during the day and, unless these add up to at least an hour, the occupation should be classified as moderately active. Individuals vary widely in the efficiency with which they perform similar tasks. For these reasons only very general guidance can be given for the energy needs of different occupations, which for this purpose can be usefully classified into three groups, as follows:

Sedentary. Men engaged in sedentary occupations for 8 hours need about 900 kcal. Such people are office workers, drivers, pilots, teachers, journalists, clergy, doctors, lawyers, architects and shop workers.

Moderately active. Men doing such work for 8 hours spend about 1200 kcal. This would apply to most of those engaged in light industry and assembly plants, to railway workers, postmen, joiners, slaters, plumbers, bus conductors and most farm workers, builders' labourers and unskilled labourers.

Very active. Men doing very active work for 8 hours spend about 1800 kcal. Work of this kind would be done by coal miners, steel workers, dockers, forestry workers, army recruits and some farm workers, builders' labourers and unskilled labourers. Mot *women*, working in the home, an office or light industry, would require about 900 kcal for an 8 hour day. Those whose work involved a great deal of physical activity might need up to 1,200 kcal.

RECREATION

The amount of energy required for recreational and non-occupational activities can vary from about 800 to about 1,800 kcal during the remaining 8 hours of the day. However, it is unlikely that this will be related to a man's occupation, and an average value of 1,300 kcal may be taken as representative of the three classes of occupation given above. For women, the corresponding value is 900 kcal.

THE DAY'S NEEDS FOR ENERGY

Summarizing the previous sections, the total daily energy expenditure of men engaged in different occupations can be set out as shown below. This total expenditure represents what should be provided each day from the food. Again, it should be emphasized that these are average values, for groups of men.

Occupation:	*Sedentary*	*Moderately active*	*Very active*
Energy expenditure:			
in bed (kcal/8 hr)	500	500	500
at work (kcal/8 hr)	900	1,200	1,800
non-occupational (kcal/8 hr)	1,300	1,300	1,300
Energy requirement:			
from food (kcal/24 hr)	2,700	3,000	3,600

For most women, the total energy requirement is about 2,200 kcal. Recommended intakes for children of various ages are given in the table on page 42.

As an example, a bank clerk may distribute his energy expenditure over a day as follows:

	kcal	kcal/day
8 hours rest in bed:		500
8 hours at work:		
5 hr mostly sitting, at 1·5 kcal/min:	450	
3 hr standing, walking etc., at 2·5 kcal/min:	450	
		900
8 hours non-occupational activities:		
1 hr washing, dressing etc., at 3·5 kcal/min:	210	
1 hr walking, at 4·2 kcal/min:	250	
4 hr sitting, at 1·4 kcal/min:	340	
1½ hr gardening, at 5·0 kcal/min:	450	
½ hr washing dishes at 1·7 kcal/min:	50	
		1,300
Total		2,700

FOOD AND FATNESS

If more food is eaten than is needed for an individual's daily activity some of it will be converted in the body into fat. Just as energy is supplied by either carbohydrate, fat or protein, so can any of these three nutrients be converted into body fat if they are eaten in excess of the energy output. Thus, the most 'fattening' foods are those which contain the most energy. These are the concentrated foods containing little water and high proportions of carbohydrate and fat such as pastry, suet pudding, sweet cakes or sweets.

Individuals differ in their tendency to form fat, but the reasons for this are not fully understood. Activity and appetite are contributory factors. In general, if people wish to lose weight they can do so by decreasing the energy value of the food eaten without changing their physical activity or by increasing their physical activity without increasing the energy value of food eaten or by a combination of the two methods.

These two principles reversed apply equally to people who want to gain weight.

In considering this matter it is important to remember the figures given in the course of this Section. For example, if a man who is trying to reduce his weight goes for a brisk half hour walk, he expends about 150 kcal. If at the end of his walk he is thirsty and drinks a pint of mild beer, the beer puts back the energy he has used up. He cannot therefore be surprised if his weight does not change. This does not mean that regular exercise is not an important factor in controlling weight.

STARVATION

During a period of starvation or severe food shortage the majority of people will lose between 15 per cent and 35 per cent of their body weight; few people can survive a weight loss of more than 35–40 per cent. In spite of the adaptation which occurs with low calorie intakes, the capacity to accomplish physical work decreases as the fat stores of the body become exhausted. It has been estimated that after about 40 days without food the energy reserves in a well-fed man will be used up and death will occur.

MECHANICAL EFFICIENCY OF THE BODY

The amount of mechanical work which a man can do in riding a bicycle or carrying bricks up a ladder can be measured and expressed in calories or joules. When the amount of work done is compared with the energy value of the food used up in doing that work, and both are expressed in the same units, the mechanical efficiency of the body can be calculated.

In the course of ordinary industrial work, the efficiency of the body is about 15 per cent. That is to say, food containing 1,600 kcal is used up when a man does 240 kcal of physical work.

As the body can convert only about 15 per cent of the energy derived from food into mechanical work (the percentage varies slightly for different kinds of mechanical effort), the remainder is converted to heat. That is why physical exercise makes the body hot.

HOT FOODS AND THE SIGNIFICANCE OF THEIR TEMPERATURE

The heat of hot food is trifling compared to the day's energy requirements. This is shown in the following example. An average soup provides 10 kcal per oz. A half-pint serving (10 oz) therefore contributes 100 kcal. The heat provided by the hotness of the soup, with a temperature of, say, 60°C, to the body, the temperature of which is 37°C, can be roughly calculated as follows:

10 oz=280 g; 1 kcal=by definition the heat needed to raise 1,000 g of water 1°C.

Hence, the heat liberated when 280 g of soup cools from 60°C to 37°C, i.e.: through 23°C, amounts to $\frac{23 \times 280}{1,000} = 6$ kcal.

It can be seen that the heat of the soup, 6 kcal, is insignificant compared with the 100 kcal in the energy value of the soup or compared with 3,000 kcal needed during the day by a moderately active man. Nevertheless, this heat warms the body in the same sort of way as would a hot-water bottle.

PART II

Inorganic Elements

THE body contains a score or so of inorganic elements, commonly called *minerals*, which must be derived from food. Eight of these are present in relatively large amounts, and 9 or more, essential for normal metabolism, are needed in much smaller quantities and are known as *trace elements* or trace minerals. These substances are used for four main purposes:

1. As constituents of bones (i.e., the rigid structures which support the muscular system of the body) and teeth. Some of these minerals are: calcium, phosphorus and magnesium.

2. As constituents of body cells, of which muscle, blood corpuscles, liver, etc., are composed. Minerals having this function include iron, phosphorus, sulphur and potassium.

3. As soluble salts which give to the body fluids their composition and stability which are both essential for life. Among elements which serve this purpose are: sodium, potassium and chlorine.

4. As factors involved in chemical reactions in the body, including those concerned with the release of energy during metabolism; for example, iron, phosphorus and magnesium.

Some of the other minerals have special purposes in the body. Iodine is a constituent of the hormone made by the thyroid gland, which plays a part in controlling the rate at which energy is used in maintaining the body processes; cobalt is a constituent of vitamin B_{12}.

Many minerals are needed only in small amounts and are widely distributed in foods. Although knowledge of their functions in the body is necessary for an understanding of nutrition, the importance of considering them in practical dietetics is small. Care must be taken, however, to ensure that two minerals, calcium and iron, are present in adequate amounts. These will be discussed later in more detail.

SODIUM

All body fluids contain salt (sodium chloride) and it is essential for life that the normal concentration of sodium chloride in the blood should be maintained. If there is a shortage of salt, muscular cramps will result.

Salt is lost from the body in two ways: in the urine, and in the sweat. The amount of salt eliminated in urine is regulated by the kidneys, but there is no means of control over the amount of salt lost in sweat, although there is evidence that during adaptation to hot climates sweat becomes more dilute and so less salt is lost in this way. Extra salt may, therefore, be needed in hot climates if adaptation is not complete; it is necessary when work is done at high temperatures, e.g., by miners in deep pits, stokers, steel workers; and after strenuous exercise. The salt requirements of the body are closely related to its water requirements.

In a temperate climate the daily amount of salt needed by an adult not doing active work is about 4 g. The whole of this may, however, be lost in sweat during three hours' exercise in the sun. People usually eat about 5–20 g daily in their food. The amount not needed in healthy persons is harmlessly eliminated in the urine. Low salt diets are useful in the treatment of certain diseases.

Besides the salt added to meals in cooking or at the table, salt is present in most foods.

Sodium content of certain foods

	mg per 100 g	mg per oz
Bacon	1,220	348
Haddock, fillet, smoked	1,220	348
Cornflakes	1,050	298
Kippers	990	281
Cheese, Cheddar	612	174
Bread, white	540	153
Peas, canned	260	74
Butter	223	63
Eggs	135	38
Herring	130	37
Beef	69	20
Milk	50	14
Peas, fresh	1	Trace

POTASSIUM

Potassium behaves chemically in a similar manner to sodium. In the body, however, sodium is present in the free fluids, but potassium is chiefly in the fluids within the cells, e.g., of the muscles and the red corpuscles of the blood. There is a loss of potassium in urine at the rate of about 2–4 g a day, which closely reflects the dietary intake. Potassium, unlike sodium, is not lost in sweat. Most common foods contain potassium, so that there is little likelihood of any deficiency in normal diets. However, old people who eat little food may obtain insufficient, especially if purgatives are frequently used.

Potassium content of certain foods

	mg per 100 g	mg per oz
Prunes, dried	864	246
Potatoes, raw	568	161
Brussels sprouts, raw	515	146
Mushrooms	467	133
Cauliflower	408	116
Beef	334	95
Liver	325	92
Herring	317	90
Haddock fillet, fresh	302	86
Bacon	250	71
Grapefruit	234	66
Milk	160	46
Eggs	138	39
Cheese, Cheddar	116	33
Cornflakes	114	32
Bread	100	28

CALCIUM

Calcium has three main functions in the body. It is necessary for:

1. Proper development and growth of bones and teeth;
2. Normal clotting of blood;
3. Normal functioning of muscles.

The Need for Calcium in Different Groups

Children who are growing and forming new bones and teeth, need more calcium than adults. If their diet does not provide enough the results are: reduced growth; rickets; and badly formed teeth.

Expectant and nursing mothers require more calcium than other adults; the expectant mother in order to form the bones of the child, and the nursing mother to provide calcium in her own milk. If insufficient calcium is available in the mother's food she will draw on that stored in her own bones.

Other adults require calcium to replace the small daily losses. However, there is no evidence that the loss of bone that accompanies advancing age can be prevented by increasing calcium intake.

Calcium in the Blood and Muscles

A small, constant proportion is present in the blood, being necessary as part of the clotting mechanism, and also for the proper functioning of muscles.

In order that the amount of calcium in the blood shall remain constant, the bones act as a reservoir from which calcium can quickly be obtained, and in which excess calcium can be deposited. The parathyroid gland, a small organ attached to the thyroid gland in the neck, controls the level of calcium in the blood. Should the parathyroid become diseased or damaged, the amount of calcium in the blood may fall. A condition of tetany (muscular spasm) will then occur, and may quickly prove fatal. Calcitonin, a hormone secreted by the thyroid and adjacent glands, and vitamin D, also regulate the level of calcium in the blood.

Calcium content of certain foods

	mg per 100 g	mg per oz		mg per 100 g	mg per oz
Dried, skimmed milk	1,277	362	Cabbage, raw	65	18
Cheese, Cheddar	810	230	Eggs	56	16
Sardines	409	116	Wholemeal bread	28	8
Evaporated milk	290	82	Fish, white	25	7
Liquid milk	120	34	Beef	10	3
White bread*	100	28	Potatoes, raw	8	2

* Includes fortification

Main sources of calcium in the diet are milk, cheese, bread and flour (if fortified) and green vegetables.

Few foods contain much calcium. Unless the diet includes enough of those which contain substantial amounts it may provide too little calcium for health. These foods are: cheese, milk and milk products; fish of which the bones are eaten (e.g., sardines, tinned salmon) and green vegetables. A source of calcium other than food is provided by water used for drinking or cooking, provided that it is 'hard' water (see also page 60).

Absorption of Calcium

The amount of calcium that the body will absorb from the diet depends on several factors. The body is able to adapt itself to wide ranges in calcium intake, and normally less than half is absorbed. Vitamin D assists absorption from the gut. The amount of phosphorus in the diet was once thought to influence calcium absoprtion, but it is unlikely that the effect is appreciable in man.

Substances that interfere with calcium absorption include phytic acid and oxalic acid, which form insoluble salts with calcium. Phytic acid occurs mainly in the bran and outer layers of cereals. Oxalic acid occurs in small quantities in some green leafy vegetables, but in large quantities in rhubarb and spinach only. However, these factors are of little practical significance, because much of the phytic acid present in bread made with yeast is broken down in baking, and neither rhubarb nor spinach is eaten in very large quantities.

Very large amounts of fat in the intestine, as can occur in some diseases, may prevent the body from obtaining calcium from food, because calcium forms salts with fat which cannot be absorbed.

Calcium Content of the British Diet

Before 1939 the British diet was thought to be short of calcium. It was feared that the changes in the composition of the national diet necessitated by the war, particularly the increased consumption of roughage and the higher extraction rate of flour, might reduce the amount of calcium absorbed from the food. To guard against calcium deficiency calcium carbonate was (and still is) added to flour.

IRON

Most of the iron in the body is present in haemoglobin, which gives blood its red colour. Haemoglobin is necessary for the transport of oxygen from the lungs to the tissues, and a sufficient supply of iron in the diet is therefore essential to health. Iron is also present in the muscle pigment myoglobin, concerned too with oxygen transport, and in enzymes involved with biological oxidations inside cells (see page 2).

Once iron is absorbed by the body, it is lost only very slowly. The haemoglobin which contains the iron is present in the red blood corpuscles, which have a life of about 120 days. At the end of that time the corpuscles break up and the iron is released; it does not escape from the body, but is used again for the formation of fresh corpuscles. These new blood cells are produced in the marrow of the bones. In spite of the fact that iron is used over and over again, its replacement from food is necessary because it may be lost in two ways: by the general wear and tear of the body and in the remains of the digestive juices passed out in faeces; and when bleeding occurs. Women therefore have a greater need than men for iron.

If food provides insufficient iron to replace the body's losses, anaemia will eventually result; but it must be emphasized that anaemia may be due to many other causes as well as to iron deficiency, and that if it is to be quickly cured, very much larger amounts of iron must be taken than can be conveniently supplied in food. These large amounts are best given medicinally as iron salts.

Apart from food, iron may be obtained from water used for cooking or drinking; from iron utensils; from wine; from curry powder, and from certain earths. In some parts of the world these may make significant—even excessive—contributions.

Iron content of certain foods

Animal foods	mg per 100 g	mg per oz	*Plant foods*	mg per 100 g	mg per oz
Liver	13·9	3·9	Cocoa powder	14·3	4·1
Kidney	13·4	3·8	Apricots, dried	4·1	1·2
Beef, corned	9·8	2·8	Bread, wholemeal	3·0	0·9
Beef, fresh	4·0	1·1	Bread, white*	1·8	0·5
Eggs	2·5	0·7	Cabbage, raw	1·0	0·3
			Wine, red	0·8	0·2
			Potatoes, raw	0·7	0·2

* Includes fortification

Main sources of iron in the diet are bread, flour and other cereals, meat, potatoes, green vegetables and eggs.

Absorption of iron

The mechanism by which iron is absorbed is very delicate and absorption normally occurs only when the body needs iron. Vitamin C assists the absorption of iron, and phytic acid, as with calcium, interferes. The availability of iron from different foods varies widely, and the effect of some foods in a mixed diet on the absorption of iron from other foods can be considerable. Iron in animal foods tends to be more available than that in vegetable foods, while some forms of inorganic iron are very poorly absorbed. Generalizations will be difficult until more research has been done.

OTHER MINERALS

PHOSPHORUS, in combination with calcium, forms most of the hard structure of bones and teeth. It is present in nearly all foods, and dietary deficiency is not known in man.

MAGNESIUM forms part of the composition of bones and teeth. It is also essential for normal metabolism. It is present in practically every type of food, and there seems no chance of its deficiency in any diet.

SULPHUR is obtained in the diet in combination with other nutrients. In particular, certain proteins are of nutritional importance because of their sulphur content: sulphur is a constituent of the amino acids methionine and cysteine. If an appropriate choice of proteins is made the amount of sulphur needed by the body will almost certainly be obtained.

IODINE is needed in only very small quantities by the body, but these amounts are essential. Iodine in the diet is derived chiefly from sea fish and shell-fish, and vegetables grown where soils contain iodine.

In some parts of America, in Switzerland and elsewhere, the soils (and hence the drinking water and the native vegetables) are deficient in iodine and there is, in consequence, a deficiency in the diet. Under such conditions cases of goitre are liable to occur among the population. The use of iodized salt has proved a good preventive measure in these areas; the problem is not always a simple one because of the presence of goitrogens in members of the Brassica family and in some other foods.

FLUORINE is found in bones and teeth. The contribution from foods and drinks, with the exceptions of tea and fish containing edible bones, is small but it is present in varying degrees in drinking water in different districts of

Great Britain. The consumption of a small amount of fluorine in the drinking water decreases the amount of dental caries in children: a concentration of 1 part per million of fluoride in drinking water is recommended. Excessive amounts, however, cause brown and white pigmentation, known as 'mottling', to occur on teeth.

OTHER TRACE ELEMENTS essential for human nutrition are copper, zinc, manganese, cobalt, selenium, molybdenum and chromium. No deficiencies are likely in Britain. Strontium is present in bones and teeth but has no known physiological function.

Vitamins

UNTIL the beginning of the twentieth century it was assumed that the diet would be adequate if sufficient protein, fat, carbohydrate and inorganic elements were supplied. This view was changed when it was shown that natural unrefined foods contain substances essential for life and health which the body is unable to form for itself. These organic substances were called vitamins and were found to be present in very minute amounts in foods. Some of the vitamins, i.e., A, D, E and K, are found mainly in fatty food and are called fat-soluble vitamins; the others, i.e., the vitamins of the B group and vitamin C, are soluble in water. This classification is primarily of historical interest. As the vitamins became identified and given chemical names it was realized they had quite distinct structures and functions.

VITAMIN A

Vitamin A occurs in certain fats and in the fatty part of some foods.

Vitamin A

1. is necessary for the growth of children;
2. plays a part in the way the eyes perceive light;
3. protects the surface tissues, particularly moist areas, such as the front of the eyes, and the lining of the respiratory tract, throat and bronchial tubes.

Sources of Vitamin A in the Diet

The chemical name of vitamin A is *retinol*. This substance is found in animal foods such as liver, dairy produce and eggs. Vegetable foods, notably carrots, contain the deep yellow pigment *carotene*; this can be converted in the body to retinol and therefore is a source of vitamin A activity. Carotene is less easily absorbed from most foods than retinol. The most convenient way of expressing the total vitamin A activity of a diet is as *retinol equivalents*. By definition, 1 μg retinol equivalent is equal to 1 μg of retinol or 6 μg of β-carotene. This equivalence takes into account the lesser availability to man of carotene, compared with retinol.

Amounts of vitamin A are still frequently measured in *international units* (i.u.) 1 i.u. of vitamin A is equal to 0·3 μg of retinol or 0·6 μg of carotene. These quantities were shown to be biologically equivalent in rats under certain special conditions. But under normal conditions in man they are not equivalent: in Britain it has been conventional to say that on average 1 i.u. of retinol is equivalent to 3 i.u. of carotene. Other conventions have been used elsewhere.

In the British diet about two thirds of the total retinol equivalents are provided by retinol itself, and one third by carotene.

Vitamin A content of certain foods

Animal foods	µg retinol per 100g	µg retinol equivalents per oz
Halibut liver oil, B.P.	900,000	255,000
Cod liver oil	22,740	6,450
Liver, ox	6,000	1,700
Butter	710	282*
Margarine	900	255†
Cheese, Cheddar	320	120*
Eggs	300	85
Herring	45	13
Milk	30	11*
Sardines	30	9

Vegetable foods	µg carotene per 100 g	µg retinol equivalents per 100 g	µg retinol equivalents per oz
Carrots, mature	12,000	2,000	567
Spinach	6,000	1,000	284
Apricots, dried	3,600	600	170
Watercress	3,000	500	142
Tomatoes	700	117	33
Cabbage	300	50	14
Peas, fresh	200	50	14

* Includes the contribution from carotene.

† As retinol only; some margarines contain carotene.

Main sources of vitamin A in the diet are butter, margarine, liver, green vegetables and carrots.

Fish liver oils are by far the most concentrated natural sources of vitamin A. At one time they were used for the fortification with vitamin A of such foods as margarine in which vitamin A does not naturally occur. Since 1954, synthetic retinol or carotene has been used increasingly to fortify margarine. The value required is 760 to 940 international units per ounce; this is equal on average to about 900 µg retinol per 100 g.

The dairy products, milk, butter, cheese and eggs may vary in the amount of vitamin A they contain; this depends on the amount in the food of the cow or hen. The concentration is usually highest in the summer when green grass is available. In milk and its products most of the vitamin A activity is provided by retinol, but some by carotene, which in such foods can for practical purposes be regarded as available as retinol.

In green vegetables the amount of carotene is proportional to their greenness. Dark green plants, such as watercress, contain greater concentrations of carotene than paler vegetables, such as cabbage. In cabbage, there is more carotene in the dark outer leaves than in the pale inner heart. In carrots the amount of carotene is proportional to their yellowness.

Both retinol and carotene are stable to ordinary cooking methods, but some loss may occur in frying. Much of the vitamin A potency is lost in sun dried fruits and in other dried foods if precautions are not taken to prevent oxidation during storage.

The body can store vitamin A in the liver, so that a large amount of vitamin eaten in the autumn can help to maintain the body adequately for some time during the winter. The high vitamin A value of liver as a food results from the use of this organ for storage by the animal or fish from which the liver was taken.

An excessively great intake of retinol can be harmful, but a large amount of carotene is not harmful although it may cause yellowing of the skin.

VITAMIN D

Vitamin D is concerned in the absorption and laying down of calcium and phosphorus in bones, and is therefore of special importance to infants and children whose bones are in the process of growth and development, and to expectant mothers in whom the bones of a foetus are developing.

When insufficient vitamin D is present in the diet of children and infants, rickets may occur.

It is important that infants should not be given too much vitamin D. A happy medium must be struck between sufficient to prevent rickets and an excess which can have other ill-effects.

Sources of Vitamin D

The body obtains vitamin D from two distinct sources: *food* and *sunlight*. Relatively few foods contain vitamin D. Those that do so naturally are all animal products. Quantities are expressed in international units or in micrograms: 1 i.u. = 0·025 μg ($\frac{1}{40}$ μg) of the pure compound cholecalciferol, or vitamin D3. The amounts present in some common foods are shown below:

Vitamin D content of certain foods

	μg per 100 g	μg per oz		μg per 100 g	μg per oz
Cod liver oil	217·50	61·66	Eggs	1·50	0·43
Herring and Kipper	22·25	6·38	Butter	1·25	0·36
Salmon, canned	12·50	3·54	Liver	0·75	0·21
Milk, dried, whole, fortified	8·83	2·50	Cheese, Cheddar	0·35	0·10
Margarine	8·00	2·27	Milk, dried, whole	0·30	0·09
Sardines, canned	7·50	2·13	Milk, liquid, summer	0·05	0·01

Main sources of vitamin D in the diet are margarine, fatty fish, eggs and butter.

There is a seasonal variation in the vitamin D content of milk, butter and cheese; in summer, dairy produce contains more vitamin D than in winter. However, the vitamin D content of fresh milk, even in summer, is insubstantial, whereas fortified dried milk is a good source of vitamin D. Herrings contain more vitamin D during the breeding season. Vitamin D is added to margarine.

Sunlight acting on the skin can cause the formation of vitamin D in the body itself. Thus, if children receive sufficient sunlight on their bodies the amount of vitamin D they will need from their food will be very much reduced, maybe to zero.

Needs of Adults for Vitamin D

Although infants, children and expectant mothers have by far the greatest need of vitamin D, other adults probably require a small amount. If there is inadequate exposure to sunlight and, in addition, the diet does not contain vitamin D, adults may develop osteomalacia, a disease of the bones bearing some similarity to rickets. These conditions are likely to be met most frequently among the elderly.

Nature of Vitamin D

Vitamin D is not soluble in water. Like vitamin A, it occurs only in fats and the fatty parts of foods. Vitamin D is comparatively resistant to heat and to the conditions likely to occur in cooking and handling food.

VITAMIN E

Vitamin E, or tocopherol, was first identified as a substance necessary for the normal fertility of rats. There is no conclusive evidence that vitamin E plays any part in influencing fertility in human beings, or that it is effective in other conditions for which it has been used. However, it is essential for normal metabolism; although it acts as an antioxidant, preventing the oxidation of certain substances in foods, it may not function in this way in the body.

It is found in small amounts in many foods; vegetable oils, wheat germ, some margarines and eggs contain larger amounts.

VITAMIN K

Vitamin K is essential for normal clotting of blood. It is found in green vegetables such as cabbage and in green peas. It can also be synthesized by bacteria in the gut. Deficiency of this vitamin is unlikely in a healthy person.

THE VITAMIN B GROUP

The vitamin B group comprises a number of substances often, but not always, found together in the same foods. These vitamins act as cofactors in enzyme systems (see page 3). The individual members of the group to be considered here are:

Thiamine, also called vitamin B_1

Riboflavine, once called vitamin B_2

Nicotinic Acid, sometimes called niacin, especially in the United States.

Besides these three substances, at least five others are known to be essential in human nutrition, and are discussed briefly: *Folic Acid*, *Vitamin* B_{12}, *Pyridoxine or vitamin* B_6, *Pantothenic Acid*, and *Biotin*. It is unlikely that a dietary deficiency of only one B vitamin would occur, and clinical symptoms would probably reflect a multiple deficiency. Unlike vitamins A and D, the vitamins in the B group cannot be stored in the body.

THIAMINE (VITAMIN B_1). Thiamine, like all the other members of the vitamin B group, is soluble in water. It is unstable at high temperatures and, consequently, a considerable amount may be lost in cooking and during the canning and processing of certain foods. It is destroyed by alkali so that food cooked with bicarbonate of soda, such as scones, usually contains little thiamine; it is also destroyed by sulphite which may be used during some processing of vegetables and fruits. Losses of thiamine during frying pre-peeled potato chips which have been dipped in sulphite solution may be 3–4 times greater than from untreated tubers.

The function of thiamine in the body is to form part of the chemical process by means of which a steady and continuous release of energy is obtained from carbohydrate.

The signs of ill-health which develop if insufficient thiamine is provided by the diet are a check in the growth of children, and development of a special type of neuritis; the subject becomes depressed, irritable and quarrelsome. Extreme deficiency results in the disease beriberi, seldom seen in Europe but common in the Far East, if people live largely on white rice from which most of the thiamine has been removed during its preparation.

The amount of thiamine needed in the diet is related to the amount of carbohydrate it contains. For practical purposes, however, it is convenient to relate requirements of thiamine to the total energy intake, and the recommended intake of thiamine is 0·04 mg per 100 kcal. To decide, therefore, whether any particular food is or is not a useful source of thiamine in the diet, it is necessary to calculate whether it provides more than 0·04 mg for each 100 kcal. For example:

(*a*) *Wholemeal bread:* 1 oz provides 68 kcal and contains 0·07 mg of thiamine. Hence sufficient wholemeal bread to provide 100 kcal also provides 0·10 mg of thiamine. This is in excess of the 0·04 mg required, so wholemeal bread contributes thiamine to the diet.

(*b*) *Pre-war white bread:* 1 oz provided 69 kcal and contained 0·02 mg of thiamine. Hence sufficient pre-war white bread to provide 100 kcal contained 0·03 mg of thiamine. This was less than the 0·04 mg needed by the body. This type of white bread was therefore deficient in thiamine and constituted a drain on the diet.

(*c*) *Present-day white bread:* 1 oz provides 72 kcal and contains 0·05 mg of thiamine, as thiamine is now added to white flour. Hence, sufficient white bread to provide 100 kcal contains 0·07 mg thiamine. This is greater than the 0·04 mg required, so white bread is now a useful source of thiamine in the diet.

If similar calculations are made, it will be found that most natural foods, including potatoes, green vegetables, milk and dairy produce, all add some thiamine to the diet. Almost the only carbohydrate food now deficient in thiamine is sugar. As thiamine is water-soluble it does not occur in fats but it is widely distributed in other foods; examples are shown in the table opposite.

In the manufacture of beer, grain is mashed in water, sugar is added and the mixture is fermented with yeast. The yeast, which is a living organism, absorbs the thiamine from the grain; therefore brewers' yeast is a particularly good source of this vitamin. It does not, however, absorb riboflavine or nicotinic acid to the same extent and consequently beer contains quite substantial amounts of these vitamins.

Thiamine content of certain foods

	mg per 100 g	mg per oz		mg per 100 g	mg per oz
Dried brewers' yeast	18·40	5·22	White bread*	0·18	0·05
Pork	1·00	0·28	Potatoes	0·11	0·03
Cornflakes	0·60	0·17	Beef	0·07	0·02
Oatmeal	0·50	0·14	Milk	0·04	0·01
Bacon	0·40	0·11	Sugar	Nil	
Peas, green	0·32	0·09	Corned beef	Nil	
Wholemeal bread (100 per cent extraction)	0·24	0·07			
Peanuts, roasted	0·23	0·07			

* See page 46.

The main sources of thiamine in the diet are bread and flour, meat, potatoes and milk.

RIBOFLAVINE. Riboflavine is a yellow substance which, like other vitamins of the B group, is soluble in water. It is not easily destroyed by heat alone, but it is destroyed by a combination of heat and ultra-violet light.

The function of riboflavine is to form a link in the chain of processes by which the body obtains energy from food.

When insufficient riboflavine is provided by the diet, the following symptoms occur:

(*a*) growth of children is checked;
(*b*) cracks and sores appear in the skin at the corners of the mouth;
(*c*) the tongue becomes magenta in colour and sore;
(*d*) the transparent front of the eyes may become misted.

Riboflavine content of certain foods

	mg per 100 g	mg per oz		mg per 100 g	mg per oz
Dried brewers' yeast	3·68	1·04	Eggs	0·35	0·10
Liver	3·00	0·85	Beef	0·20	0·06
Cheese	0·50	0·14	Milk	0·15	0·04

The main sources of riboflavine in the diet are liquid milk, meat, particularly liver, and eggs.

To avoid riboflavine losses, milk in bottles should not be exposed to sunlight (see also page 33).

NICOTINIC ACID. Nicotinic acid is soluble in water but stable to heat at normal cooking temperatures. It is converted to its active form, nicotinamide, in the body. This substance is also formed from the amino acid tryptophan. Therefore the body's needs may be supplied from both these sources. For this reason it is convenient to express nicotinic acid in terms of equivalents: by definition, 1 *mg nicotinic acid equivalent is equal to* 1 *mg of available nicotinic acid or* 60 *mg of tryptophan.*

The function of nicotinic acid is to form another link in the chain of processes by which the body obtains energy from food.

When there is insufficient nicotinic acid in the diet the following signs of ill-health occur:

(*a*) growth of children is checked;
(*b*) the skin becomes rough and red, especially where exposed to the light, as on the face, hands and neck;

(*c*) the tongue becomes red and sore;
(*d*) diarrhoea and other signs of digestive upset appear;
(*e*) mental symptoms develop such as dementia or confusion;
(*f*) in severe cases the disease pellagra develops, in which the above symptoms are aggravated.

The nicotinic acid and tryptophan contents of some foods are shown below. As a useful generalization, animal proteins contain 1·4 per cent of tryptophan, and vegetable proteins 1·0 per cent. The nicotinic acid naturally present in cereals is not available to man, being in a bound form called *niacytin*, and so should not be included in assessing the number of nicotinic acid equivalents in a food or diet.

Nicotinic acid equivalents in certain foods

	Nicotinic acid (total) mg/100 g	Tryptophan mg/100 g	Nicotinic acid* equivalents mg/100 g	Nicotinic acid* equivalents mg/oz
Dried brewers' yeast	53·4	552	62·9	17·8
Liver	13·0	248	17·1	4·9
Beef	5·0	168	7·8	2·2
Fish, white	3·0	179	6·0	1·7
Cheese, Cheddar	0·1	306	5·2	1·5
Peas, fresh	2·5	58	3·5	1·0
Eggs	0·1	177	3·0	0·9
Bread, wholemeal	2·6	116	1·9†	0·5†
Bread, white	1·4	105	2·3‡	0·7‡
Potatoes	1·2	34	1·8	0·5
Milk	0·1	47	0·9	0·3

* Available nicotinic acid plus $\frac{\text{tryptophan}}{60}$

† From tryptophan only.
‡ From tryptophan and added nicotinic acid.

Main sources of nicotinic acid equivalents in the diet are meat and meat products, bread, flour, other cereals, vegetables and fruit, and milk.

FOLIC ACID. This term is commonly used for a variety of related substances with different biological activities. Folic acid is concerned with the synthesis of nucleoproteins. Deficiency causes megaloblastic anaemia, sometimes found in infants, the elderly and in pregnancy. It occurs in many foods, particularly liver and leafy green vegetables.

VITAMIN B_{12}. Vitamin B_{12} is the most recently discovered member of the B group and, unlike other vitamins, it contains a metal—cobalt. It is probably part of at least one enzyme system involved in the metabolism of protein, fat and carbohydrate and, with folic acid, of nucleic acids. It is necessary for growth, the prevention of certain sorts of anaemia, including pernicious anaemia, and the prevention of degeneration of nerve cells, particularly of the spinal cord. It is only found in foods of animal origin; liver is the richest source but it is also present in milk, meat, eggs and fish.

PYRIDOXINE. Pyridoxine, also called vitamin B_6, is necessary for the growth of all young animals. It is concerned with several enzyme systems involved in metabolism, particularly in the breakdown and synthesis of tryptophan and other amino acids. It is also concerned with fat metabolism, red blood cell formation, the nervous system and the health of the skin. Yeast, liver, cereals and pulses are the best sources, but it is present in smaller amounts in most foods.

PANTOTHENIC ACID. This is also concerned with the health of the skin and with growth and with antibody production. It is associated with enzyme systems involved in the metabolism of fat and carbohydrate. It is widely distributed in foods, but is found in larger amounts in yeast, liver, kidney, egg yolk and cereals.

BIOTIN. Biotin is necessary for the health of the skin and probably forms part of several enzyme systems in metabolism. In raw egg white there is a substance called avidin which inhibits the action of biotin so that, if large quanties of raw egg white are eaten, symptoms of illness may occur. Cooked egg white does not have this effect. Egg yolk, liver, kidney and yeast are the richest sources, but it is present in a wide variety of foods. Biotin can be synthesized by bacteria in the intestine, and may not be necessary in the diet.

VITAMIN C (ASCORBIC ACID)

In applying the science of nutrition to the practical planning of diets care must be taken to ensure an adequate supply of vitamin C. A proper supply of all vitamins is necessary for an adequate diet, but in many cases individual substances are so widely distributed, and required by the body in such small amounts, that no problem of supply arises.

For example, vitamin A (retinol) is present in animal foods, such as dairy produce and eggs, and carotene in vegetable foods, such as greens and carrots. Thiamine is found in almost all foods where it is needed, except sugar. It is therefore not difficult to design a diet containing enough of these two nutrients, even though this is not always done.

The two facts which make it easy for a diet to be insufficiently provided with vitamin C are:

(*a*) Vitamin C occurs almost entirely in vegetable foods, i.e., fruit and vegetables which are sometimes in short supply and expensive. The few animal foods in which it occurs, i.e., fresh liver, fresh meat and milk, contain only very small amounts.

(*b*) Vitamin C may easily be destroyed by cooking. With green vegetables, for example, even if the best methods are used, it is difficult to avoid losing at least half the amount originally present. (See also page 58).

Vitamin C is concerned in a complex way with the structure of connective tissue. If insufficient vitamin C is provided by the diet, certain ill-effects will arise. The growth of children will be checked. Apart from this, little becomes manifest until the subject is near to the point of scurvy. Then stresses lead to pathological conditions, for example, bleeding around the hair follicles, infected gums, failure of wounds or fractures to heal. Later frank scurvy supervenes.

Vitamin C is very easily soluble in water. In plants, however, the vitamin is enclosed within the cells. In these cells is also found an enzyme, a substance which works with the vitamin in carrying on the life of the plant. When plant cells are destroyed, either by cooking or by mechanical means such as grating or mincing, the ordered life of the plant is disrupted and the enzyme destroys the vitamin C. This destruction can be minimized by destroying the enzyme itself (see page 59).

Vitamin C content of certain foods

	mg per 100 g	mg per oz
Black currants	200	57
Brussels sprouts, raw	100	28
Cauliflower, raw	70	20
Cabbage, raw	60	17
Strawberries	60	17
Oranges	50	14
Lemons	50	14
Grapefruit	40	11
Potatoes, raw:		
New	30	9
October, November	20	6
December	15	4
January, February	10	3
March onwards	8	2
Tomatoes	20	6
Lettuce	15	4
Apples, plums, pears	3–5	1

The main sources of vitamin C in the diet are potatoes, green vegetables and fresh citrus fruits.

The amount of vitamin C in raw fruits and vegetables is very variable even within the same variety; the values given above are broadly representative.

In green vegetables the amount of vitamin C is highest in the spring and early summer when the plants are making rapid growth. For example, brussels sprouts and spring cabbage may contain 50 or 60 mg of vitamin C per oz, if they are harvested when they are growing most quickly. When vegetables begin to wilt, either due to long storage or other causes, vitamin C is rapidly lost.

As can be seen from the Table, the vitamin C in potatoes decreases during storage. The concentration is highest in late summer when the crop is lifted and thereafter steadily falls during the winter and spring. Although the amount of vitamin C in an ounce of potato is never as high as that in many other foods, potatoes may be the principal source of vitamin C in the diet because they are often eaten every day in quite large amounts. Before potatoes were introduced into Europe, scurvy was a common disease at the end of every winter.

Although black currants, and next to them oranges, lemons and grapefruit, are among the richest common sources of vitamin C, higher concentrations have been discovered in less common fruits. For example, rose hips may contain up to 700 mg of vitamin C per oz, i.e., 2·5 per cent of the fruit consists of vitamin C. The average figure for rose hips is about 170 mg per oz. Hips cannot be eaten as such, because the fine hairs surrounding the pips irritate the digestive tract. Syrups and other forms of extract can, however, be made from them.

Seeds, including cereal grains and, it is important to note, dried peas and beans, contain no vitamin C. When seeds are sprouted, however, vitamin C is produced. In circumstances where normal sources of vitamin C are unavailable, ill health can be avoided if dried peas or grains are moistened, allowed to sprout, and then eaten in that form.

Vitamin C in Milk

A baby can derive enough vitamin C from its mother's milk provided the mother's diet is good. Cow's milk, which soon becomes an important item in the infant's diet, contains a small amount of vitamin C. It is, however, wise dietetic practice to start giving orange juice or some other suitable source to infants at an early age as a safeguard, because cow's milk is not a dependable source. Milk left on the doorstep for half an hour, will have lost at least half of its vitamin C before it is consumed. This reaction is initiated by the riboflavine in the milk which is also destroyed.

Needs of Animals for Vitamin C

If the human diet does not contain vitamin C, health will suffer and finally scurvy will develop. The need for vitamin C is not, however, shared by all animal species. Although guinea-pigs and monkeys, like man, need vitamin C to protect them against scurvy, rats and other animals can synthesize the vitamin and need no dietary source.

PART III

Digestion of Foods and Absorption of Nutrients

FOOD has been defined as anything, either solid or liquid, which, when swallowed, can supply the body with energy; enable the body to grow; or participate in the mechanisms regulating the body functions. Food can do none of these things until it is absorbed. While a piece of bread remains in the mouth, it has not fulfilled any of the functions of food until, at least, it has been swallowed. Indeed, substances can travel further than the mouth without necessarily being absorbed. For example, after poison has reached the stomach it can still be recovered if an emetic is given quickly enough. It can thus be said that:

While nutrients remain in the digestive tract they are not properly in the body and can fulfil none of their functions as essential components of food.

It follows that if food has exerted an influence on the body, whether it be the supply of energy, the stimulation of growth or the regulation of function, it must have been absorbed.

The body itself, in which the processes of life are found, includes the head, the limbs, the skeleton, the blood system and all the parts through which blood flows. Within the body lies the digestive tract, which is, in spite of many elaborations, a tube open at both ends:

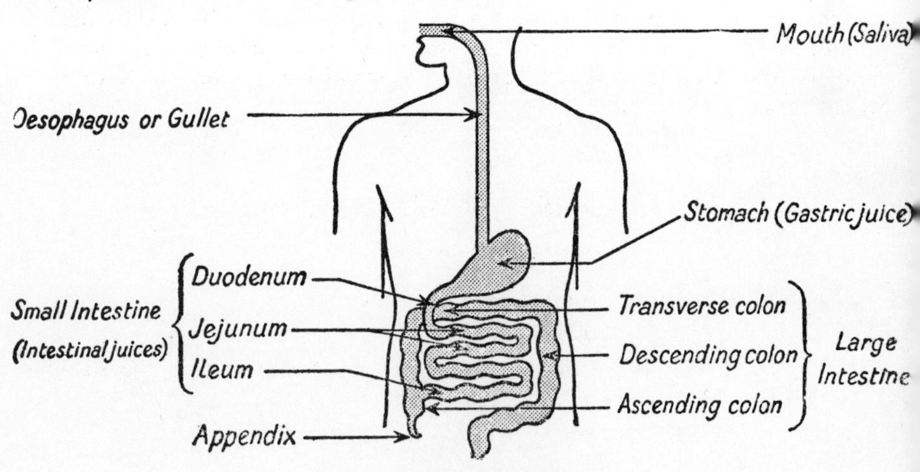

Diagram of Digestive System

Only when digested food has passed through the moist walls of the digestive tract into the blood beyond can it be said to have passed into the body.

Digestion. Before the nutrients in food can enter the bloodstream, most foods must be broken down into their component parts by digestive juices and by the mechanical action of the teeth and the muscular movement of other parts of the digestive tract. This process of breakdown is digestion.

Absorption. This is the process by which separate nutrients and their breakdown products pass into the walls of the digestive tract and thence into the blood. Only after absorption can the body derive benefit from food.

APPETITE, FLAVOUR AND DIGESTION

Appetite. When the stomach is empty and the body is short of energy, hunger pains, due to muscular contractions of the stomach, may make themselves felt, and there is a desire to eat. The sensation of *hunger* is also produced by changes in the amounts of certain nutrients in the blood. Appetite is a different sensation which relates to particular foods and is influenced by the surroundings and emotional state of the eater. The appetizing smell of food causes a flow of saliva and gastric juice and the desire to eat, even if there is no cause for real hunger. Meat and some other foods contain extractives which, although they themselves may have almost no food value, aid these processes.

Thus, if meals are attractive and appetizing and contain 'extractives' there will be a flow of juices and the food will be easily digested. On the other hand, the following conditions will reduce the amount of juices and consequently cause delay and difficulty in digestion: unpleasant appearance or smell of the food, and worry, fear or anger before or during eating.

Tasty food and nutrition. Although tasty food stimulates the flow of digestive juices and encourages people to eat, it does not follow that food which people dislike does not nourish them too, provided they eat it. Indeed, in certain circumstances it is necessary to supply nutrients by means of a stomach tube. Nevertheless, where the individual has a free choice, attractive food has the important nutritional significance of being more likely to be eaten.

PROCESS OF DIGESTION

THE MOUTH

(*a*) Food is mechanically broken down by chewing.

(*b*) It is mixed and moistened with saliva.

(*c*) The saliva breaks down a small amount of starch into the sugar maltose.

Saliva

This is derived from the salivary glands in and under the tongue and in the mouth. Thoughts of food, and the smell and taste of food, cause it to flow. After food has been chewed and mixed with saliva in the mouth, it is swallowed and passes into the stomach.

The Stomach

(*a*) More mixing and mechanical breakdown occurs,

(*b*) About 3 litres (2–3 quarts) of gastric juice are produced each day by a normal stomach. This juice, for the performance of its work, contains 0·2 to 0·4 per cent of hydrochloric acid. By the action of gastric juice:

(i) proteins are partly broken down;

(ii) milk is coagulated in preparation for digestion.

Gastric Juice

This is derived from the stomach itself; it flows into the stomach when saliva flows into the mouth. Besides hydrochloric acid, gastric juice contains the enzyme pepsin which acts specifically to split protein.

Speed of Digestion in the Stomach

Different foods stay in the stomach for different lengths of time, generally between two and four hours; the lower end of the stomach then opens and allows the now semi-liquid food to pass by degrees into the small intestine.

While it is commonly considered that foods which pass quickly through the stomach are more readily digested than those which do not, it is not necessarily an advantage for food to leave the stomach rapidly, because the more quickly the stomach empties the sooner will hunger be felt again.

Fats eaten with other foods possess the power of delaying the passage of those foods through the stomach; for this reason fats are said to possess a high *satiety value*.

The Small Intestine

The small intestine is a tube about an inch in diameter and about 20 feet long, divided and named thus:

(*a*) The first 12 inches of intestine nearest the stomach are called the *duodenum* (from the Latin *duodenum digitorum* meaning space of twelve fingers' breadth). Intestinal juices enter the intestine in the duodenum.

(*b*) The next 9 feet of intestine are called the *jejunum* (*jejunus* is Latin for 'empty': the jejunum is usually found to be empty after death).

(*c*) The final 9 or 10 feet of the small intestine make up the *ileum* (*eileos* is Greek for 'twisted').

Food is moved down the whole length of the intestine by rhythmic muscular contraction of the gut walls. Absorption occurs all along the route. About four hours after a meal is eaten the final residue begins to be passed in liquid form, through a valve which prevents any reverse movement, into the large intestine.

Intestinal Juices

(*a*) The effect of the acid mixture from the stomach on the walls of the intestine causes a substance called secretin to be passed into the blood. The secretin is carried by the circulation of the blood to the *pancreas*, an organ connected by a duct (or tube) to the duodenum.

When the secretin reaches the pancreas it causes a digestive juice to be secreted which passes into the duodenum. This juice is alkaline and neutralizes the acid mixture from the stomach. It contains a variety of enzymes, notably trypsin, amylase and lipase, which act respectively on protein, starch and fat.

(*b*) Bile also enters the duodenum from the gall bladder, having been made in the liver. Bile emulsifies fat so that it can be chemically split by the digestive juice from the pancreas.

(*c*) A third juice, the intestinal juice, is derived from the walls of the small intestine itself.

With the aid of these juices:

(i) Starch is broken down to glucose, and sucrose to glucose and fructose.

(ii) Proteins, partly digested in the stomach, are further broken down to their final units, amino acids.

(iii) Fats are emulsified and most are split into glycerol and fatty acids.

The Large Intestine

Some substances reached the large intestine undigested. A small amount of nutrients may be freed by bacteria from otherwise indigestible material, such as cellulose. In the process bacteria use them for their own food and can synthesize certain vitamins, notably some of the B group and vitamin K. It is uncertain how much of the products are available to the body.

The large intestine is a tube about 2 inches in diameter and about 5 feet long. The first part, on the right side of the body where the faeces travel up, is the *ascending colon*. The portion passing across the body from right to left is the *transverse colon*, and the last main portion on the left side of the body, where the faeces travel down, is the descending colon. Faeces are finally expelled from the large intestine through the *anus*. It is quite normal for faeces to leave the body 24 hours or more after the meal from which they were derived.

Process of Absorption

THE MOUTH. Very little is absorbed into the body through the lining of the inside of the mouth.

THE STOMACH. The following substances pass in small quantities through the lining of the stomach into the blood stream:

alcohol; sugar; mineral salts which are soluble in water, e.g., common salt; vitamins which are soluble in water, e.g., vitamins of the B group and vitamin C; water.

THE SMALL INTESTINE. By far the greater part of the absorption of all nutrients takes place in the small intestine: i.e., the products of digestion of dietary carbohydrate, protein and fat, and the remains of the digestive juices, and minerals, and vitamins.

THE LARGE INTESTINE. Very little absorption of nutrients occurs in the large intestine. The principal function of the large intestine is to absorb water from the indigestible residue of foodstuffs which go to form the faeces.

Absorption of Water

When water or watery liquids (such as soft drinks) are drunk, about one-fifth is absorbed into the blood through the stomach and the remaining four-fifths through the small and large intestines. If an excess of water is absorbed, sufficient to dilute the blood, enough will be withdrawn by the kidneys to maintain the correct composition of blood. This automatic control by the kidneys is so sensitive and rapid that within an hour or less of drinking fluid in excess of the body's needs, the water will have been eliminated through the kidneys.

The Fate of Nutrients in the Body

CARBOHYDRATES. These are partly broken down by saliva in the mouth; they pass through the stomach and are finally split up into monosaccharides (see page 5) in the small intestine. Thence they pass into the blood. The digestibility of carbohydrate in a normal mixed diet is about 98 per cent. Any indigestible cellulose or similar material passes on into the large intestine.

The blood stream carries sugars derived from food to the liver, where they are stored as glycogen (see Blood Sugar, page 39). Glycogen is also stored in the muscles. When the body needs energy, the glycogen is converted back to glucose. Glucose may also be converted into fatty acids, which are stored in the body as fat, or used by the tissues as a major source of energy.

During the course of physical activity, glucose is used up by the muscles. Supplies are consequently transferred by the blood from the liver to the muscles to take the place of the glucose expended.

FATS. Fats pass unchanged through the mouth and the stomach. In the intestine, however, fat is finely divided into small droplets until it is completely emulsified, split into its component parts by the digestive juices, (see page 37) resynthesized into triglycerides in cells of the intestinal wall, and absorbed into the lymph in which it is carried until it enters the blood stream. When in the blood stream, the majority of the fat from food is laid down in the body's fat depots, from which it may be constantly utilized. The rest is brought to the liver and muscles where some of it may be used, together with carbohydrate, for the production of energy. The average digestibility of fat is 95 per cent.

PROTEINS. These pass through the mouth unchanged. They are partly broken down in the stomach, and the process is finally completed in the small intestine, where absorption of amino acids takes place. The digestibility of protein in a mixed diet is about 92 per cent.

The amino acids pass through the wall of the small intestine into the blood and are carried to the liver and other tissues, where they mix with the amino acids derived from the normal continuous breakdown of body proteins to form a 'metabolic pool'. The amino acids in this pool can take part in a great number of chemical reactions, including the synthesis of body proteins, nucleic acids and some hormones. The body has a very limited ability to store amino acids. Those (the majority) that are not used in the above processes are used for the production of energy. In this event the nitrogen contained in amino acids is removed in the liver and converted into urea, which is eliminated by the kidneys. Having lost their nitrogen, the amino acids contain only carbon, hydrogen and oxygen, and can be used as fuel. If the pattern of the amino acids in the pool is not well suited for the synthetic reactions to take place (see page 10), or if the total energy intake is inadequate for the body's needs, then still more of the amino acids in the pool are used for energy purposes.

MINERALS. Soluble salts, such as salts of *sodium* and *potassium*, are readily absorbed by the stomach and the small intestine. Salts of this nature, surplus to the body's needs, are eliminated by the kidney.

Calcium is absorbed in the small intestine. The proportion of calcium in foods which is unavailable to the body travels through the large intestine and is lost with the faeces. About 20 per cent of the calcium in the diet is normally absorbed, but this proportion depends on many factors, including the customary intake of calcium.

Iron is only absorbed by the body when required. It passes into the blood through the walls of the small intestine and excess (unabsorbed) leaves the body by the large intestine. The availability of iron in different foods has already been discussed (see page 23).

VITAMINS. The *water-soluble vitamins* of the B group and vitamin C are absorbed in the stomach and the small intestine. Only a small quantity of these can be stored in the body. If more is taken than needed to saturate the blood, the excess is eliminated by the kidneys.

The *fat-soluble vitamins* A and D are absorbed only in the small intestine. Absorption may not occur if the digestion of fats is poor. Excess of these vitamins can be stored in the liver and only in exceptional circumstances is any lost in the urine.

BLOOD SUGAR

When any kind of carbohydrate is digested, it is ultimately converted into glucose, in which form it is passed into the blood. The composition of the blood, which must be steadily maintained if life is to continue, normally includes a small amount of glucose. The blood glucose is essential as brain cells can only use glucose as a source of energy. Muscle cells and other tissues also use glucose directly, but much if not most of their energy is derived from free fatty acids in the blood.

When a normal individual eats carbohydrate, the glucose formed from it in the intestine causes a slight rise in the level of blood sugar. This, however, is soon reduced, as the hormone insulin, passed into the blood by the pancreas, causes the withdrawal of glucose into the cells of muscles and other tissues. In the condition of *diabetes* there is a deficiency of insulin and the concentration of glucose in the blood rises steadily until at last it spills over, through the kidneys, and is lost in the urine.

Another hormone, adrenaline, which is produced by two glands, the adrenals, situated close to the kidneys, has an opposite effect to insulin. It causes a withdrawal of glucose from the liver and a consequent rapid rise in the concentration of glucose in the blood, e.g., when a man is angry or frightened. The increase of sugar in the blood provides fuel for immediate and violent physical action should the reason for the anger or fear demand it.

Still other hormones are involved in the control of blood glucose, which is maintained at a relatively constant level despite wide variations in food intake and tissue utilization.

Recommended Nutrient Intakes

FOR health and efficiency an individual must have a sufficient intake of all the nutrients so far discussed. However, there is no nutritional advantage or benefit to health in having an intake above an individual's requirements of any nutrient. These essential nutrients are present in varying proportions in different foods and it is therefore possible to design an adequate diet in a number of ways to suit local tastes and diverse food supplies; to be satisfactory any diet must contain adequate amounts of all the nutrients.

Because individuals vary widely in their requirements it is usually impracticable if not impossible to discuss what these are; therefore, a number of judgements have been made by national and international bodies, on the best evidence available, of amounts of the different nutrients that will satisfy the needs of most people. Such amounts are commonly referred to as nutritional or dietary allowances, or recommended intakes.

The figures given in Table 1 on page 42 are those recommended by the Department of Health and Social Security in a report published in 1969. The recommended intakes of nutrients are defined as the amounts sufficient or more than sufficient for the nutritional needs of practically all healthy persons in the categories specified. They are thought to be sensible and practicable for the United Kingdom now but, like all such recommendations, they are liable to revision in the light of new knowledge or change of circumstances.

The recommendations may be used as guides in the planning and interpretation of diets. But if a diet does not fulfill the recommendations this fact does not in itself constitute evidence of malnutrition.

ENERGY. It has been made plain that sufficient food to meet energy requirements must be consumed if physical work is to be done and vigour and weight retained over a long period. If too much food is consumed the excess will be stored as fat, while if too little is eaten, and physical activity continues, the body will become thin. Individuals vary widely in their energy needs, and the recommended intakes of energy are equal to average energy requirements, so that they do not refer to individuals but only to groups. Recommended intakes of energy are given both in kilocalories and in megajoules (see page 3).

PROTEIN. The recommended intakes of protein given on page 42 are somewhat arbitrary values, representing 10 per cent of the energy requirement; they are based more on considerations of a palatable diet, and the provision of other nutrients, than on the strict physiological need for protein. There is evidence that man can consume much smaller quantities, of a similar quality to that of the usual British diet, and still retain good health. If energy requirements are not fully met the protein that is eaten will not be efficiently utilized: in this situation protein nutrition will be improved only by increasing the energy intake.

FAT. There appears to be no hard and fast nutritional requirement for fat, apart from the need for a small amount of the essential fatty acids (see page 8). On present evidence this need amounts to 1 to 2 per cent of the energy requirement, and British diets supply much more than this. In Britain, 40 per cent of the energy value of the average diet is provided by fat. Some authorities consider this excessive, but the proportion could not fall below 30 per cent without radical changes in dietary habits. If the diet is lacking in fat it will tend to become very bulky, since fat is the most compact and concentrated of all sources of energy. Fat is also of great value in making a diet varied.

THIAMINE. The amount of thiamine necessary varies with the energy requirement: the recommended intake is 0·4 mg per 1,000 kcal. Most foods contain sufficient thiamine per 1,000 kcal, with the notable exception of sugar; but as this vitamin is water-soluble it is not present in fats extracted from either vegetable or animal sources. For example, there is sufficient in milk, but practically none in butter.

RIBOFLAVINE. The recommended intake is related to the cell mass of the body. The figures in Table 1 are, however, based on the recommendation of a Joint Committee of the Food and Agriculture Organization and the World Health Organization in 1967 for moderately active adult men and women. Current evidence does not suggest that the riboflavine requirements of the elderly are less than those of younger adults although cell mass decreases. The distribution of riboflavine in foods is not so uniform as that of thiamine.

NICOTINIC ACID. The recommended intake is likewise based on the FAO/WHO recommendation for moderately active men and women. The use of nicotinic acid equivalents recognizes the fact that tryptophan can be converted in the body to nicotinic acid (see page 29).

VITAMIN C. There are differing opinions as to the quantity of vitamin C required for health. It is generally agreed that 10 mg daily will prevent and cure scurvy. The recommended intake of 30 mg daily for adults is thought to provide a reasonable safety margin. The National Research Council of the United States of America recommends 60 mg daily for adult men, basing their estimates on different criteria.

VITAMIN A. The figures in Table 1 are given in *micrograms of retinol equivalents*, instead of in the more familiar international units. The recommendations may be met either from retinol (vitamin A), found in animal foods; or from its precursor carotene, found in vegetable foods, which has on average one sixth (by weight) the activity of retinol; or of course from combinations of both. For further details see page 24.

VITAMIN D. It is not possible to make firm estimates of the dietary need for vitamin D because this vitamin can be formed in the skin by the action of sunlight. The amounts recommended may be thought of as a safety measure, but those who are housebound and not exposed to sunlight, such as the elderly, may need more. Amounts of 2·5 μg, equivalent to 100 i.u., have been successfully used to treat elderly patients with osteomalacia.

TABLE 1

Recommended Daily Intakes of Energy and Nutrients for the UK (Department of Health and Social Security, 1969)

(a) Age range	Occupational category	(c) Body weight	(d) Energy		(f) Protein	(g) Thiamine	Ribo-flavine	Nicotinic acid	Ascorbic acid	Vitamin A	(j) Vitamin D	Calcium	Iron
		kg	kcal	(e) MJ	g	mg	mg	(h) mg equivalents	mg	(i) µg retinol equivalents	µg cholecal-ciferol	mg	mg
BOYS AND GIRLS													
0 up to 1 year (b)		7·3	800	3·3	20	0·3	0·4	5	15	450	10	600(l)	6(l)
1 up to 2 years		11·4	1,200	5·0	30	0·5	0·6	7	20	300	10	500	7
2 up to 3 years		13·5	1,400	5·9	35	0·6	0·7	8	20	300	10	500	7
3 up to 5 years		16·5	1,600	6·7	40	0·6	0·8	9	20	300	10	500	8
5 up to 7 years		20·5	1,800	7·5	45	0·7	0·9	10	20	300	2·5	500	8
7 up to 9 years		25·1	2,100	8·8	53	0·8	1·0	11	20	400	2·5	500	10
BOYS													
9 up to 12 years		31·9	2,500	10·5	63	1·0	1·2	14	25	575	2·5	700	13
12 up to 15 years		45·5	2,800	11·7	70	1·1	1·4	16	25	725	2·5	700	14
15 up to 18 years		61·0	3,000	12·6	75	1·2	1·7	19	30	750	2·5	600	15
GIRLS													
9 up to 12 years		33·0	2,300	9·6	58	0·9	1·2	13	25	575	2·5	700	13
12 up to 15 years		48·6	2,300	9·6	58	0·9	1·4	16	25	725	2·5	700	14
15 up to 18 years		56·1	2,300	9·6	58	0·9	1·4	16	30	750	2·5	600	15
MEN													
18 up to 35 years	Sedentary	65	2,700	11·3	68	1·1	1·7	18	30	750	2·5	500	10
	Moderately active		3,000	12·6	75	1·2	1·7	18	30	750	2·5	500	10
	Very active		3,600	15·1	90	1·4	1·7	18	30	750	2·5	500	10
35 up to 65 years	Sedentary	65	2,600	10·9	65	1·0	1·7	18	30	750	2·5	500	10
	Moderately active		2,900	12·1	73	1·2	1·7	18	30	750	2·5	500	10
	Very active		3,600	15·1	90	1·4	1·7	18	30	750	2·5	500	10
65 up to 75 years	Assuming a sedentary life	63	2,350	9·8	59	0·9	1·7	18	30	750	2·5	500	10
75 and over		63	2,100	8·8	53	0·8	1·7	18	30	750	2·5	500	10
WOMEN													
18 up to 55 years	Most occupations	55	2,200	9·2	55	0·9	1·3	15	30	750	2·5	500	12
	Very active		2,500	10·5	63	1·0	1·3	15	30	750	2·5	500	12
55 up to 75 years	Assuming a sedentary life	53	2,050	8·6	51	0·8	1·3	15	30	750	2·5	500	10
75 and over		53	1,900	8·0	48	0·7	1·3	15	30	750	2·5	500	10
Pregnancy, 2nd and 3rd trimester			2,400	10·0	60	1·0	1·6	18	60	750	10(k)	1,200(m)	15
Lactation			2,700	11·3	68	1·1	1·8	21	60	1,200	10	1,200	15

Footnotes

(a) The ages are from one birthday to another: e.g., 9 up to 12 is from the 9th up to, but not including, the 12th birthday. The figures in the Table in general refer to the mid-point of the ranges, though those for the range 18 up to 35 refer to the age 25 years, and for the range 18 up to 55, to 35 years of age.

(b) Average figures relating to the first year of life. Energy and minimum protein requirements for the four trimesters are given elsewhere in the DHSS report.

(c) The body weights of children and adolescents are averages and relate to London in 1965.
The body weights of adults do not represent average values; they are those of the FAO reference man and woman, with a nominal reduction for the elderly.

(d) Average requirements relating to groups of individuals.

(e) Megajoules (10^6 joules). Calculated from the relation 1 kilocalorie = 4·186 kilojoules, and rounded to 1 decimal place.

(f) Recommended intakes calculated as providing 10 per cent of energy requirements. Minimum protein requirements given in Table 3 of the DHSS report.

(g) The figures, calculated from energy requirements and the recommended intake of thiamine of 0·4 mg/1,000 kcal, relate to groups of individuals.

(h) 1 nicotinic acid equivalent = 1 mg available nicotinic acid or 60 mg tryptophan.

(i) 1 retinol equivalent = 1 µg retinol or 6 µg β-carotene or 12 µg other biologically active carotenoids.

(j) No dietary source may be necessary for those adequately exposed to sunlight, but the requirement for the housebound may be greater than that recommended.

(k) For all three trimesters.

(l) These figures apply to infants who are not breast fed. Infants who are entirely breast fed receive smaller quantities; these are adequate since absorption from breast milk is higher.

TABLE 2

Recommended Intakes of Nutrients* per 1,000 kcal (Derived from recommendations of the Department of Health and Social Security 1969)

Category		Minimum protein requirement	Riboflavine	Nicotinic acid	Ascorbic acid	Vitamin A	Vitamin D	Calcium	Iron
		g	mg	mg equivalents	mg	µg retinol equivalents	µg	mg	mg
BOYS AND GIRLS									
0 up to 1 year		19	0·50	6·3	19	560	12·5	750	7·5
1 up to 2 years		16	0·50	5·8	17	250	8·3	420	5·8
2 up to 3 years		15	0·50	5·7	14	210	7·1	360	5·0
3 up to 5 years		16	0·50	5·6	13	190	6·3	310	5·0
5 up to 7 years		16	0·50	5·7	11	170	1·4	280	4·4
7 up to 9 years		14	0·48	5·2	10	190	1·2	240	4·8
BOYS									
9 up to 12 years		14	0·48	5·6	10	230	1·0	280	5·2
12 up to 15 years		16	0·50	5·7	9	260	0·9	250	5·0
15 up to 18 years		17	0·57	6·3	10	250	0·8	200	5·0
GIRLS									
9 up to 12 years		15	0·52	5·7	11	250	1·1	300	5·8
12 up to 15 years		19	0·61	7·0	11	320	1·1	300	6·1
15 up to 18 years		17	0·61	7·0	13	330	1·1	260	6·5
MEN									
18 up to 35 years:	Sedentary	17	0·63	6·7	11	280	0·9	190	3·7
	Moderately active	15	0·57	6·0	10	250	0·8	170	3·3
	Very active	13	0·47	5·0	8	210	0·7	140	2·8
35 up to 65 years:	Sedentary	17	0·65	6·9	12	290	1·0	190	3·9
	Moderately active	15	0·59	6·2	10	260	0·9	170	3·5
	Very active	12	0·47	5·0	8	210	0·7	140	2·8
65 up to 75 years: }	Assuming a sedentary life	17	0·72	7·7	13	320	1·1	210	4·3
75 and over: }		18	0·81	8·6	14	360	1·2	240	4·8
WOMEN									
18 up to 55 years:	Most occupations	17	0·59	6·8	14	340	1·1	230	5·5
	Very active	15	0·52	6·0	12	300	1·0	200	4·8
55 up to 75 years: }	Assuming a sedentary life	18	0·63	7·3	15	370	1·2	240	4·9
75 and over: }		18	0·68	7·9	16	400	1·3	260	5·3
Pregnancy, 2nd and 3rd trimester		18	0·67	7·5	25	310	4·2	500	6·3
Lactation		20	0·67	7·8	22	440	3·7	440	5·6

*For all categories, the recommended intake of dietary protein is 25 g per 1,000 kcal and of thiamine is 0·4 mg per 1,000 kcal.

CALCIUM. The figures in Table 1 are based on a FAO/WHO report of 1962. The recommended intakes for children are up to 700 mg of calcium daily, an amount that would be provided by 1 pint of milk. Milk is rich in calcium and therefore particularly valuable in children's diets.

IRON. Because of uncertainties about the absorption of iron (see page 23) it is difficult to assess dietary requirements with any precision. The recommendations in the Table represent a reasonable guide for mixed diets as eaten in the United Kingdom. Younger women have a greater need for iron than men, since they suffer from a periodical loss of blood.

The recommended intakes of nutrients are set out in Table 2 (page 43) in another form, in terms of the recommendations for energy; in practice it is the intake of energy that determines the intake of nutrients.

AN ADEQUATE DIET

In this section precise amounts of energy and of nine nutrients needed for an adequate diet by all types of individuals, from infants to active workers, have been suggested. Other nutrients also have dietary importance, but the report of the Department of Health and Social Security (1969) made no detailed recommendations for these, although for some of them an attempt to do so was made by the National Research Council of the United States in the most recent revision (1968) of its Recommended Dietary Allowances.

Despite the lack of figures for these other nutrients, adequacy of the diet can be safeguarded by the inclusion of as wide a variety of foods as possible (see also page 65).

Synthetic vitamin C can be added to a diet calculated to be lacking in it, but is better supplied in oranges (or other suitable fruits), salads and other vegetables. If these foods are used, some at least of the other nutrients may be supplied as well.

Deficiency of some nutrients is felt more quickly than a deficiency of others. Shortage of energy is immediately felt as hunger, but if the diet has previously been well balanced and adequately supplied with protein and other nutrients, newly imposed shortages of specific nutrients will not manifest themselves for some months.

In practice, diets are not often found to be deficient in only one nutrient. Deficiency of vitamins of the B group may cause a sore tongue and cracks at the corners of the mouth. These can be symptoms of riboflavine deficiency; if, however, pure riboflavine is given the tongue and mouth may be cured but severe dermatitis of the face and hands may develop. These are symptoms of nicotinic acid deficiency. It sometimes happens that sufferers have been eating a diet deficient in all B-vitamins and that the symptoms of only one deficiency occur. If that deficiency alone is treated, symptoms of one of the others may appear. The correct treatment is to provide a diet fully adequate in all nutrients.

Composition of Food

The detailed composition of food in terms of nutrients is given in Appendix A (page 75) and should constantly be referred to in the course of this section.

THE figures are expressed per 100 g and per ounce of the raw, edible portion of each food, unless otherwise indicated. A table is also included in which the nutrient content of foods is expressed in terms of their energy content, i.e., per 100 kcal. This table can usefully be compared with Table 2 on page 43 which shows the recommended intake of nutrients expressed per 1,000 kcal.

The contribution that a food can make to the diet depends not only on its nutrient content, but also on the quantity in which it is eaten. Table 3 on page 52 shows the contributions of different foods to the nutrient content of the average diet in Great Britain, and—in conjunction with Appendix A—will indicate the relative nutritional importance of various foods. When using tables of food composition it is important to remember that variations occur between different samples of the same food, and that the figures given in any food table are representative values. It is essential to understand what the figures imply. They may be expressed, as in most of Appendix A, in terms of the composition of the *raw* '*edible portion*', or they may have been adjusted so that they relate to the *gross weight of food* including inedible material, when they are usually called '*as purchased*' values. In other words, in 'as purchased' tables the weight of food includes such inedible material as bones, rind or skin, but the composition figures given relate to the chemical composition of the edible portion included in the weight as purchased.

For example, the energy value of potatoes given in Appendix A is 22 kcal per oz of raw, edible potato. Wastage in potatoes varies from 7 per cent when new, to 25 per cent when old. If 75 per cent of the weight of old potatoes 'as purchased' is edible, then the energy value of 1 oz of old potato as purchased would be:

$$\frac{75}{100} \times 22 = 17 \text{ kcal (to the nearest whole number)}$$

A third method of expression is to give the chemical composition of the *cooked edible portion* which is usually termed '*as served*'. Such values take into account changes in weight and losses of nutrients on cooking.

Directions for use are given with most tables of food composition. It is important to follow such directions when calculating the nutritive value of food.

CEREALS

All the common cereals (wheat, oats, barley, rye, maize, rice, etc.) are principally sources of carbohydrate. The amount of available carbohydrate in the whole grain varies from about 66 per cent (oats) to 72 per cent (rye). Compared with this, protein can range from 8 per cent (rice) to 14 per cent (Canadian wheat), and fat from just over 1 per cent (rye, barley and rice) to 6 per cent (oats). Cereal grains contain approximately 13 per cent of moisture.

With the application of the techniques of plant breeding to the production of new varieties of cereals, their composition, particularly their protein content, is changing. This must be borne in mind, and the facts checked, when the nutritive value of diets containing high proportions of cereals is being considered.

In flour milling the term 'extraction rate' means the percentage of flour which is separated from a given weight of wheat. This can be varied according to the type of flour required, giving, for example, white, brown, or wholemeal flours.

If the whole grain is ground as flour the product is called 100 per cent extraction flour, i.e., true wholemeal.

Brown flours contain a proportion of the tough outer coats of the grain. These contain both indigestible fibre, which reduces the digestibility of the flour, and phytic acid, which may combine with some of the calcium in the diet and prevent its absorption by the body. This is not of great practical importance.

White flours consist mainly of the innermost part of the grain, i.e., the endosperm. The distribution of nutrients within the wheat grain is not uniform; the concentration of protein and vitamins is higher in the germ and outer layers of the grain than in the inner starchy endosperm. As the extraction rate of flour rises the digestibility falls, but the disadvantages have to be considered in relation to the nutritional advantages. These are: more protein; more iron; and more vitamins of the B group. In this context it should be noted that nicotinic acid in cereals occurs in a bound form which is normally unavailable to man; cereals or cereal products to which nicotinic acid has been artificially added will, however, contribute towards the daily intake of the vitamin.

It is possible to devise experiments with rats that demonstrate the nutritional superiority of wholemeal flour, but the rats must be very young and the diets must contain an abnormally high proportion of flour. It has not been possible to demonstrate these differences with children. In Britain, where a wide variety of food is commonly eaten, nutritional differences between wholemeal and fortified white flours are not likely to have any practical significance.

To safeguard the nutritional value of bread and flour, the Government has, in the course of time, instituted certain Orders and Regulations. The latest* were brought into force in September 1964 and state that all flours must contain the following minimum quantities of nutrients:

	per 100 g
Iron	1·65 mg
Thiamine (vitamin B_1)	0·24 mg
Nicotinic acid	1·60 mg

These are the levels occurring naturally in 80 per cent extraction flour. Flours of about 72 per cent extraction, as now used, have to be fortified with these nutrients to bring their concentrations to the prescribed levels.

The Regulations also require that calcium carbonate (creta praeparata) should be added to all except true wholemeal flour and self raising flour which has a calcium compound as a raising ingredient. This is done at the rate of 14 oz per 280 lb sack of flour. At the time of going to press the Bread and Flour Regulations are under review.

---

* Statutory Instrument No. 1435, 1963.

MILK is the most complete of all foods and it is also easily digested. It is particularly valuable for its contribution of calcium, riboflavine and protein to the diet, but it is comparatively deficient in iron, and vitamins C and D. Considerable losses of vitamin C and riboflavine may occur during distribution. The carbohydrate in milk is in the form of lactose (page 5). In homogenized milk the fat remains evenly distributed throughout the liquid instead of rising to the surface as cream. The composition of milk, as shown in Appendix A, will vary slightly with the breed of cow, the stage of lactation and the season of the year. The nutrients which are most affected are milk fat and vitamins A and D. Various types of milk are available both in liquid and dried forms. These will be discussed in the section on page 55.

SKIM MILK is milk from which most of the fat has been removed. It is of good nutritional value for its content of protein, calcium and riboflavine.

CREAM. This is derived from milk either by allowing the butter-fat to rise to the top or by mechanical separation. Minimum fat contents are laid down in Government Regulations.* Single cream must contain at least 18 per cent by weight of milk fat, whereas double cream contains not less than 48 per cent, compared with 3·8 per cent in milk.

YOGHURT. The nutritional value of yoghurt is essentially similar to that of the milk and minor ingredients used in its preparation. The commercial product is based either on whole milk or on skimmed milk which is innoculated with a selected culture under controlled conditions. Powdered skimmed milk may be added to produce a firmer curd; flavourings, fruit juices, fruit and sugar are sometimes incorporated to give a varied product. Some varieties of yoghurt are fortified with vitamins.

BUTTER is made from cow's milk by separation of the cream, which is then churned. Most butters contain over 80 per cent of milk fat and the maximum moisture content allowed is 16 per cent. 1–2 per cent of salt is added to salted butter during manufacture. The amounts of vitamin A and D in butter are variable; the values shown in Appendix A are representative.

CHEDDAR CHEESE. This is composed of about one-third protein, one-third fat and one-third water. As can be seen from Appendix A, it is an excellent source of calcium.

Cheeses of various types differ principally because of the different organisms used to cause coagulation of protein during manufacture. Hard cheeses, such as the Cheddar and Cheshire varieties, are, in general, of higher nutritive value than soft cheeses, such as Camembert and Gorgonzola, because they contain less moisture. Cream cheese has a high fat content. Parmesan cheese, which contains more protein than an average cheese, is made from partly skimmed cow's milk.

Certain cheeses are made from milk other than cow's milk. For example, Roquefort cheese is made from sheep's milk.

EGGS are a good source of protein and egg yolk is a good source of iron, though there is evidence that one of the proteins in egg white may hinder absorption. Eggs also provide substantial amounts of vitamins A and D and riboflavine, and small amounts of other vitamins of the B group, including vitamin B_{12}, which is not present in vegetable foods.

---

* Statutory Instrument No. 752, 1970.

MEAT

The lean part of meat, which is a valuable source of high quality protein, is made up of a number of muscle fibres. These fibres differ in length in various types of meat. They are longer in old than in young animals, they are also longer in crab, for example, than in breast of chicken.

The outer part of each fibre is made up of tough connective tissue of a gristle-like nature. When a beefsteak is pounded the muscle fibres are broken apart so that the meat is made more tender.

Deposits of fat, 'marbling', are found in spaces between the muscle fibres. Each separate muscle fibre is a tube which contains water, soluble protein, mineral salts, and extractives.

Effect of Hanging Meat. When meat is allowed to hang, acids develop which cause the muscle fibres to soften. The meat thus becomes more tender, and the acids also give it a stronger flavour. This method of softening meat is common with game.

The nutrient composition of various types of meat is shown in Appendix A. There is not necessarily more nourishment in expensive meat than in cheaper cuts, nor has frozen meat any lower value than fresh meat. Corned beef has, however, lost a proportion of its nicotinic acid and riboflavine, and contains no thiamine. Liver and kidney contain less fat than most meat. Liver, particularly, is very rich in vitamin A, and is also a very good dietary source of iron and riboflavine and other B vitamins. Sweetbreads and tripe are useful and easily digestible sources of animal protein. Tripe contains much more calcium than other meats; this is derived from the lime with which it is treated during preparation.

The fairly large variation in the fat content of all types of carcase meat will directly affect its energy content. The values in Appendix A are intended to apply to meat of average fatness.

POULTRY

Like carcase meat, poultry is a source of high quality protein; consumption is now more than three times as great as pre-war. This trend is due to the introduction of the broiler and a consequent fall in the price of poultry meat. Differences in the nutrient composition of broiler chickens and free range chickens are of no significance in a balanced diet.

FISH

The muscle of fish is as useful a source of animal protein as meat. The fat of fish, unlike fat in meat, provides vitamins A and D in the diet; it is also highly unsaturated. As can be seen in Appendix A the proportion of fat in different types of fish varies widely. Fatty fish (herring, mackerel, salmon, eel) contain from 10 to 18 per cent of fat, while white fish (cod, haddock, sole, whiting, etc.) contain less than 2 per cent in the flesh. Those fish of which the bones are eaten provide an excellent source of calcium and phosphorus. This group includes whitebait, sardines, sprats and canned salmon.

VEGETABLES

GREEN VEGETABLES. These are of nutritional importance because of their content of carotene, the precursor of vitamin A, and vitamin C. Green vegetables also contain useful amounts of iron but the extent to which this is utilized is variable (see page 23). The figures given in Appendix A are representative values; individual specimens may vary widely in composition. Vitamin C content is highest in the early summer; carotene increases in proportion with the greenness of the vegetable: the green of chlorophyll masks the deep yellow of carotene. Green vegetables provide little energy, only a trace of fat and a small amount of protein. Owing to their high water content they are bulky foods. They also contain a comparatively large amount of indigestible fibre.

ROOTS AND TUBERS. The most important of these are potatoes. When large amounts of potatoes are eaten, the amount of energy obtained is substantial. In many diets potatoes provide most of the vitamin C and useful amounts of thiamine and nicotinic acid, but the amount of thiamine will fall if pre-peeled potatoes are used (see page 59). Carrots have already been mentioned as exceptional among roots in containing a large amount of carotene, which provides vitamin A. Turnips and swedes contain vitamin C, but are otherwise of little nutritive value. They contain 91–93 per cent water, which is more than the amount found in milk.

PEAS AND BEANS. Green peas, broad beans and haricot beans contain more energy, protein and thiamine than other fresh vegetables. Green garden peas and broad beans also contain vitamin C and carotene.

Dried peas and beans must not be confused with fresh or dehydrated vegetables. The dried forms are rich in energy, protein and other nutrients. It is, however, important to remember that, before dried peas and beans can be used, they must be soaked. When this is done the moisture content rises from 12 to 70 per cent; in peas the energy value falls from 274 to 99 kcal per 100 g. They contain no vitamin C.

DEHYDRATED VEGETABLES. Raw vegetables trimmed and prepared for cooking contain 80 to 95 per cent of water; this water can be removed by dehydration, a controlled drying process which reduces the moisture content to between 5 and 10 per cent, in such a way that the qualities of the fresh vegetable are retained. Vitamin C is rather more stable in dehydrated than in fresh green vegetables, so that there will be at least as much vitamin C in a serving of cooked, dehydrated cabbage as in a similar portion of cooked fresh cabbage provided it has been stored properly i.e., its colour is green. In processed potato flakes and mashed potato powder, the loss of vitamin C can be considerable. If sulphite is added to dehydrated vegetables to preserve colour and vitamin C and to extend storage life, most of the thiamine will be destroyed.

QUICK-FROZEN VEGETABLES. The nutrients of fresh foods are generally well retained during the quick-freezing process. Vegetables are harvested immediately they reach prime condition and rapid processing leads to the maximum retention of nutrients.

FRUIT

FRESH FRUIT. When ripe, fresh fruit contains sugar which makes it sweet, but the main nutritive importance of fruit is as a source of vitamin C. In Appendix A, however, it will be seen that, except for black currants, strawberries and one or two others, fruits do not compare favourably with vegetables as sources of vitamin C.

DRIED FRUITS. Dried fruits such as currants, raisins, dates and figs provide energy, principally in the form of sugar. Prunes and dried apricots are also useful sources of carotene. Dried fruits do not contain vitamin C.

NUTS are highly nutritious. They are rich in protein and fat, and consequently are a concentrated source of energy. They contain no vitamin A or vitamin C, but are unusually rich in thiamine. Nuts are not easily digested because they contain a high proportion of tough fibres.

ALCOHOL

The alcohol in alcoholic drinks can be utilized by man as a source of energy, 1 gram of alcohol providing 7 kcal. Some alcoholic drinks, for example beer, also contain carbohydrate, and this provides additional energy. The average alcohol consumption in the U.K. provides about 100 kcal per adult per day. Chronic alcoholics may obtain a large proportion of their energy intake from alcohol, with a consequent reduction in their intake of protein and vitamins; multiple vitamin deficiencies in chronic alcoholics are thus not uncommon. The alcoholic strength of drinks in this country is shown by a *proof* measure; 70 per cent proof spirit contains 40 per cent alcohol. The alcohol content and energy value of some alcoholic drinks is shown in the table below.

	Alcohol g/100 ml	Carbohydrate g/100 g	Energy Value kcal/100 ml
Brown ale, bottled	2·2	3·0	28
Draught ale, mild	2·6	1·6	25
Strong ale	6·6	6·1	73
Cider, sweet	3·7	4·3	42
Sherry, sweet	15·6	6·9	135
Port	15·6	11·4	152
Graves	8·8	3·4	73
Burgundy	10·1	0·4	72
Spirits (70% Proof)	31·5	Tr	222

CONTRIBUTION OF DIFFERENT FOODS TO THE NUTRIENT CONTENT OF THE DIET

It has already been stated that the value of a food in the diet depends not only on its content of the various nutrients, but on the quantities in which it is normally eaten. Earlier in this section details were given of the composition of foods, and in each of the sections on the individual nutrients figures were given for the nutrient content of certain foods together with the main sources in the diet. Table 3 on page 52 shows the contribution of different foods to the nutrient content of the total diet, and thus places the importance of the various foods in perspective.

The estimates are based on the National Food Survey consumption data and are national averages for the whole of Great Britain. They vary little from year to year.

The Table shows that milk, cream and cheese supply over 60 per cent of the calcium in the diet and over 40 per cent of the riboflavine, as well as important quantities of protein, vitamins A and D, thiamine and nicotinic acid equivalents (derived chiefly from the tryptophan, see page 30). The meat group supplies a quarter of the protein and is the largest contributor to the diet of nicotinic acid equivalents; it also provides iron, vitamin A (mainly from liver) thiamine and riboflavine. The fats are principally of importance, apart from their energy value, as sources of the fat soluble vitamins A and D, margarine supplying a third of the total vitamin D. Bread and flour are the largest contributors of thiamine and supply important quantities of protein, iron, calcium and nicotinic acid equivalents. Fresh fruit is largely of value for its supply of vitamin C, but potatoes make the greatest contribution of this vitamin. Potatoes also provide useful amounts of iron, thiamine and nicotinic acid equivalents. Green vegetables are mainly of importance for their vitamin C content and root vegetables (mainly carrots) for their supply of carotene (see page 25).

Fish and eggs make small contributions to most nutrients, but are useful sources of vitamin D; eggs also contribute to the riboflavine and vitamin A content of the diet. Tea and coffee supply useful amounts of riboflavine and nicotinic acid equivalents. The only significant contribution made by sugar and preserves to the diet is to its energy value.

TABLE 3
Percentage Contribution of Different Foods to the Nutrient Content of the Average Household Diet

	Energy value	Protein	Fat	Calcium	Iron	Vitamin A (retinol equivalents)	Thiamine	Riboflavine	Nicotinic acid equivalents	Vitamin C	Vitamin D
Milk (including cream)	11	19	14	51	3	13	15	38	13	9	8
Cheese	2	4	4	10	1	4	—	4	2	—	2
Total Milk, Cream and Cheese	13	23	18	61	4	17	15	42	15	9	10
Meat, carcase	7	13	14	} 1	13	1	7	8	17	—	—
Bacon	3	3	7	}	2	—	5	2	3	—	—
Other meat	6	11	9	1	14	24	6	11	14	1	1
Total Meat	16	27	30	2	29	25	18	21	34	1	1
Fish	1	5	1	2	2	—	1	1	4	—	21
Eggs	2	5	3	2	7	7	4	8	4	—	17
Margarine	4	—	8	—	—	8	—	—	—	—	32
Butter	7	—	18	—	—	18	—	—	—	—	10
Other fats	4	—	9	—	—	—	—	—	—	—	—
Total Fats	15	—	35	—	—	26	—	—	—	—	42
Sugar and Preserves	12	—	—	—	1	—	—	—	—	2	—
Potatoes	5	4	—	1	8	—	12	3	10	31	—
Green vegetables	}	2	—	2	3	2	3	2	2	13	—
Root vegetables	} 2	—	—	1	1	15	—	—	—	2	—
Other vegetables	}	3	1	2	6	3	3	2	3	5	—
Total Vegetables	7	9	1	6	18	20	18	7	15	51	—
Fresh fruit	1	1	—	1	2	2	3	1	1	26	—
Other fruit, including nuts	1	—	—	1	2	1	1	1	1	10	—
Total Fruit	2	1	—	2	4	3	4	2	2	36	—
Bread and flour	19	21	2	18	22	—	28	4	14	—	—
Cakes, pastries, biscuits and other cereals	11	7	9	6	10	1	10	8	6	—	8
Total Cereals	30	28	11	24	32	1	38	12	20	—	8
Beverages and other food	2	2	1	1	3	1	2	7	6	1	1
Total	100	100	100	100	100	100	100	100	100	100	100

PART IV

Cooking

The Effects of Cooking and Processing on Foods and Nutrients

In the home, heat for cooking food is generally applied in one of three ways:

(*a*) Roasting and grilling: using dry heat with or without additional fat.

(*b*) Boiling, stewing and braising: in which water is used.

(*c*) Frying: in which fat is used.

In some circumstances, particularly for snack meals in hospitals or canteens, microwaves and infra-red heat may be utilized.

The application of heat brings about certain chemical and physical changes in food which, in general, improve the appearance, flavour, palatability and digestibility of the raw product and may increase its keeping quality. In this section of the Manual the effect of *cooking* on separate nutrients is discussed in general terms in relation to each main group of foods, e.g., cereals, dairy produce, eggs and meat. Variations in methods of food preparation and cooking may increase the nutritive value of the product; for example, by the addition of eggs, flour and milk in the form of a coating batter before frying; on the other hand certain culinary practices can lead to increased losses of labile vitamins. Because of such variations the nutrient composition of cooked foods is often difficult to assess accurately.

Controlled methods of *food processing*, including canning, freezing and dehydration, are applied by the food manufacturer to an increasing number of foods, which in the marketing process are transported or stored before they reach the consumer. The effects of these treatments on the nutrients in the food are also briefly discussed.

MEAT

The composition of meat has been mentioned on page 48. The myoglobin in the muscle tissues which is largely responsible for the red colour of raw meat, changes at temperatures of 65°C and above, forming the brown colour which is associated with cooked meat.

Heat causes the proteins in the muscle fibres to coagulate and the meat becomes firm, shrinkage occurs and this in turn causes extrusion of meat juices which is accompanied by loss of weight. Losses of fat and meat juices increase as the temperature rises, and the total weight loss is influenced by the cooking temperature and the internal temperature to which the meat is cooked. Variations in the proportions of muscle, fat and connective tissue in different parts of the carcase also affect weight loss. The factors that affect loss of weight of meat during cooking may, therefore, be broadly divided into two groups, those concerned with the meat itself, and those concerned with the cooking conditions. Some cheaper cuts of meat which contain a higher proportion of connective tissue will become more palatable if a slow moist method of cooking is used for their preparation, e.g., stewing or braising, which allows the collagen in the connective tissue to be converted to gelatin, thus making the meat more tender. Pressure cooking is also useful for this purpose.

The most important vitamins present in carcase meat and offal are members of the B group, mainly thiamine, riboflavine and nicotinic acid. Organs such as liver and kidney are also rich sources of vitamin A (see page 48) but only traces are present in the muscular tissue.

Vitamin A being fat soluble and relatively stable to heat, is little affected when meat is cooked unless the fat is lost. The vitamins of the B group, on the other hand, are all water soluble and will be found in the drip, stock or gravy. Thiamine is particularly sensitive to heat, and cooking losses vary between 30 and 50 per cent. Riboflavine and nicotinic acid are more stable and, as a result, the losses are smaller. The degree of destruction of folic acid which has been reported is very variable; pyridoxine and pantothenic acid are also sensitive to heat.

Microwave cooking

Present rather limited evidence suggests that the nutrient content of lean meat cooked by this method is not significantly different from meat which has been conventionally roasted. If the meat contains bone or internal areas of fat it does not heat evenly.

Processing

The loss of thiamine when meat is *canned* is generally slightly greater than in cooked meat. There is no evidence of any significant loss of nutrients from meat during *freezing*. Nutrients are also generally well retained in meat during *accelerated freeze drying*, the combined processing and cooking losses being of the same order as for the corresponding fresh meat after cooking.

The *irradiation* of food for human consumption is controlled by Government Regulations* and at present no commercially irradiated foods are sold in this country.

Meat extractives are water soluble substances from meat which include peptides, vitamins of the B group and mineral salts; they provide, with fat, most of the flavour and aroma of meat and act as a stimulant to the secretion of gastric juice.

Commercial meat extract is a by-product of corned beef manufacture. The liquid in which successive batches of meat have been heated is concentrated after removal of the fat. When the meat extract containing the dissolved solids is diluted again for consumption, the amount of protein and energy which it contributes to the soup or beverage is too small to be of importance in the diet.

Stock is made by boiling meat bones in water. The hot water extracts only a small amount of fat and gelatin from the bone marrow and a small quantity of extractives which provide the flavour. Stock is usually used as a basis for soup and it is the addition of other ingredients, e.g., milk, fat and flour in cream soups, which provide most of the nutritional value of the soup.

* Food (Control of Irradiation) Regulations 1967.

FISH

The changes that occur in cooking fish are similar to those that take place in meat, but the shrinkage is not so great. The flavour of white fish is greatly reduced by boiling, which results in a loss of approximately 40 per cent of the mineral salts. Fatty fish, such as herrings, sprats and salmon, contain vitamin A, and are a good source of vitamin D. Both these vitamins are heat-stable.

When fish is canned there may be a slight loss of thiamine and vitamin A, but otherwise smoke curing and canning have little effect on the nutrients in fish. There is no indication that modern methods of quick freezing affect the nutritive value of fish.

MILK

Partial coagulation of the proteins occurs on heating and a scum forms across the milk surface. This holds the steam and thus causes the characteristic 'boiling over'. If milk is used as a liquid in which food is cooked, e.g., fish baked in milk, the fish can cause coagulation of the milk proteins. Caramelization of the sugars in milk may occur with long cooking in a very slow oven, e.g., in milk puddings.

Most of the liquid milk supply in Great Britain is *pasteurized.* This mild form of heat treatment destroys disease-causing bacteria and causes a slight decline in nutritive value; about 10 per cent of the thiamine is destroyed and about 20 per cent of the vitamin C. Similar losses occur when milk is *spray dried.* These processes have no material effect on the nutritional value of milk as a food. *Instant skimmed milk powder* contains very little fat and therefore lacks the two important vitamins which are present in the fat, namely vitamins A and D.

Another form of heat treatment sometimes applied to milk is *sterilization.* This causes a loss of 50 per cent of vitamin C and about 30 per cent of thiamine. Sterilized milk appears thicker and creamier than fresh milk; it is homogenized before processing so that the cream does not rise to the top. *Evaporated milk* is prepared by the removal of water at low temperatures; the concentrated milk is then sterilized in cans at 116°C (240°F) which results in a loss of about 60 per cent of vitamin C and 20 per cent of thiamine. *Sweetened condensed milk* is not processed at a temperature above 100°C (212°F), and accordingly the loss of nutritive value is smaller, being about 15 per cent for vitamin C and 5 to 10 per cent for thiamine.

Milk can also be sterilized by what is known as the *UHT* (ultra-high-temperature) *process.* This involves heating the milk to about 133°C for one or two seconds. There is little change of flavour and, if the product is packed aseptically in suitable containers, it will keep for several months at room temperature. Relatively small losses of vitamins occur during the UHT treatment of milk, but there may be considerable losses of folic acid and vitamins C, B_6 and B_{12} during subsequent storage.

EGGS

When eggs are boiled or fried the proteins coagulate first in the white, at approximately 60°C (140°F), then in the yolk, between 65°C (149°F) and 68°C (154°F). The white becomes opaque and firm; the yolk thickens, then becomes dry. This property of coagulation makes eggs suitable for binding dry ingredients together in cooking, and for thickening sauces and soups; the mixture of eggs and milk completely sets in egg custard. The proteins curdle and contract slightly when over-cooked and this causes a yellow watery fluid to separate out; this may occur when scrambling eggs or boiling sauces to which eggs have been added.

When eggs are beaten, the proteins of the white especially will hold air and form a stable foam; this coagulates or sets at a very low temperature and is consequently used in the preparation of products such as meringues; eggs can also be used as raising agents, e.g., in sponge cakes, and will aid emulsification, e.g., in mayonnaise.

Iron sulphide is formed during cooking from hydrogen sulphide in the white and iron in the yolk of the egg, and this may cause blackness round the yolk in hard boiled eggs. The discoloration can be reduced by cooling the eggs in cold water immediately after cooking.

Egg white is more digestible when cooked. Hard boiled eggs are, however, slightly less digestible than those which are lightly boiled.

When eggs are cooked there is some loss of the vitamins of the B group. For example, it appears that the average loss of thiamine as a result of boiling, frying, poaching or scrambling may be between 5 and 15 per cent. Similar losses of riboflavine also occur. During frying, the fat content of eggs is increased by about 50 per cent.

CHEESE

When cheese is heated the fat melts and separates out. The proteins coagulate and shrink, and long cooking may cause stringing and toughening. With exposure to high temperatures it becomes brown. Cooking has little effect on the nutritive value of cheese.

FATS

At high temperatures fats melt and decompose into fatty acids and acrolein, and their colour darkens. Each fat decomposes at a specific temperature known as its smoking point. This is gradually lowered by cooking.

Cooking has little effect on the fat-soluble vitamins A and D. Water is driven off, and on cooling the fat tends to become more brittle.

CEREALS

Cooking is essential for the complete digestion and absorption of starch, which is by far the most important source of carbohydrate and energy in the diet. In any cereal, cooking causes the insoluble starch granules to swell up, burst and gelatinize (see page 6).

Cereals that are eaten in their natural form, e.g., rice, barley and maize, are usually prepared by boiling in water. The products of grains, e.g., flour, oatmeal and cornflour, are used in made-up foods.

Flours which will produce a large loaf of good quality are derived from 'strong' varieties of wheat; these have a slightly higher protein content than the 'weak' wheats, which provide flour suitable for making biscuits and cakes.

Thiamine is the vitamin mainly affected during the baking or processing of cereal products, because it is sensitive to heat. Riboflavine and nicotinic acid are more stable to heat and the loss on baking is small; it has already been mentioned that the nicotinic acid in cereals is not normally available to man (see page 46).

The most important factors affecting baking losses of thiamine are the final temperature and the duration of heating.

Bread

Yeast is most commonly used with flour in bread-making. This ferments part of the starch in the flour, breaking it down to alcohol, then to carbon dioxide and water which are driven off, thus causing the bread to rise. When water is added the proteins gliadin and glutenin in the flour combine to form gluten. The gluten holds the gas and then coagulates on cooking, thus holding the bread in shape. It is important that such factors as the acidity of the dough, the duration of the yeast fermentation and the conditions of baking are carefully regulated, since these affect both the production of a good loaf and the degree of destruction of phytic acid (see page 22) even in wholemeal bread.

The average amount of thiamine lost when white bread is baked is about 15 per cent.

The Chorleywood Bread Process is a new method of making bread in which the fermentation of the dough is replaced by a few minutes of intense mechanical agitation in special high speed mixers. By 1969 about two-thirds of British bread was made in this way. Experimental work has shown that breads produced by this process and by conventional methods, do not differ significantly in nutritional value.

Toast

In toasting bread, the thiamine content is further reduced. The total loss on toasting varies between 15 per cent from thick slices and 30 per cent from thin slices. However, the action of the heat drives off water, so the concentration of nutrients in terms of weight rises.

Cakes

When making a cake, such as a Madeira cake, air is held in the mixture by creaming together the fat and sugar. The eggs are lightly beaten, to incorporate air, before being added and the flour is folded in lightly so that this air is not pushed out of the mixture. When heated, the fat melts, releasing any air it may surround, and this rises through the dough. If a raising agent is used, such as baking powder, carbon dioxide is produced which enlarges the air bubbles present and swells out the starch in the flour. The starch gelatinizes and the flour and egg proteins coagulate.

The effect of baking on the nutritive value of cakes depends on whether or not bicarbonate of soda or baking powder is used. For instance, in Madeira cakes the loss of thiamine due to baking, where no raising agent was included, was found to be about 20 per cent; but where a raising agent was used, the loss of this vitamin was increased to about 30 per cent (see page 28).

Biscuits

The method of preparation is usually similar to that of cakes, but eggs are omitted. The proportion of liquid to flour is smaller in biscuits than in cakes so the starch cannot be gelatinized to the same extent.

The effect of baking on the nutritive value of biscuits is to reduce the thiamine content by 20–30 per cent. This takes into account the possible inclusion of a raising agent.

Breakfast Cereals

During the manufacture of breakfast cereals there is a loss of thiamine. In puffed or flaked products it is usually a total loss, but the manufacturing process in shredded wheat is less drastic and only between 40 and 50 per cent is lost. Some breakfast cereals are enriched with thiamine, riboflavine and nicotinic acid. When porridge is made from coarse oatmeal the cooking loss of thiamine is about 10 per cent.

VEGETABLES

The main purpose of cooking vegetables is to soften the cellular tissue and to gelatinize any starch that may be present so that it is more easily digested and absorbed. The green colour of leafy vegetables is intensified during cooking; slight over-cooking results in yellowness.

Weight changes in preparation and cooking. Peeling and trimming may reduce the purchased weight of some vegetables by one third or more (Appendix A); changes in the weight of most raw vegetables during boiling are small; in chipped potatoes there is a loss, mainly of water, of about 40 per cent.

Nutrient losses in vegetables, and to a smaller extent in fruit, are due to the passage of soluble mineral salts and vitamins from the tissues into the cooking water, and to the destruction of some labile vitamins by heat. Some vitamin C and thiamine are inevitably lost when water is used for cooking, because both these vitamins are soluble in water. It follows that the greater the volume of water used, the greater is the loss. Heat, especially prolonged heat, also destroys vitamin C and a further loss occurs if the vegetables are kept hot for any length of time. For example, after keeping hot for 30 minutes, cabbage will contain only about 60 per cent of its freshly cooked value, and the amount of vitamin C may fall to 40 per cent after one hour. This rate of loss is accelerated by the use of bicarbonate of soda.

Potatoes are an important source of vitamin C in the diet; average losses during cooking are:

	per cent
Boiled in their skins	20–40
Baked in their skins	20–40
Fried	25–35
Boiled, after peeling	30–50

In cooked potatoes, the loss of vitamin C is greater if the vegetables are mashed and then kept hot, than if they are left whole under similar conditions.

Green vegetables lose on the average about 70 per cent of their vitamin C during cooking. This is destroyed in three ways:

(1) by leaching into the cooking water;
(2) by the application of heat;
(3) by the action of plant enzymes before the temperature is sufficiently high to destroy them. This enzyme action can be minimized if vegetables are plunged immediately into boiling water at the start of the cooking process. This causes destruction of the enzymes.

Salads. The loss of approximately 70 per cent of the vitamin C in green vegetables during cooking can be almost completely avoided by eating the vegetable raw, e.g., in salad. A raw vegetable is, however, much bulkier and it is shown below that cooked greens could be a better source of the vitamin because they are normally consumed in larger quantities.

	Vitamin C mg
Average serving of lettuce (1 oz) provides	4
Average serving of raw cabbage (1 oz) provides	17
Average serving of cooked cabbage (4 oz) provides	24

Processing

Canned vegetables retain about 60 per cent of the water soluble nutrients, but one third of these are in the liquid.

Vegetables which are preserved by *quick freezing* will lose some vitamin C during the distribution and storage of the frozen food if the temperature is allowed to exceed −18°C (0°F). Correctly cooked frozen vegetables are very similar in nutritive value to cooked, fresh vegetables.

(*Dehydrated vegetables* see page 49).

The centralized preparation of *pre-peeled potatoes* for distribution to catering establishments is a comparatively recent development. The use of a sulphite dip prevents discoloration of the raw potatoes, but the amount of thiamine which is lost when the treated potatoes are boiled or fried as chips is greatly increased (see page 28).

FRUIT

The cellulose is broken down and made digestible during cooking and gums which may be present, as in plums for example, are changed to sugars, and appear in a jelly-like form.

Vitamin C, found particularly in summer fruits, such as black currants and gooseberries and in citrus fruits, is partially destroyed by cooking. The more acid the solution, the smaller this loss, and it follows that it will be less in fruits than in vegetables since most fruits are acidic.

	Vitamin C mg/100 g
Black currants (raw) contain	200
Black currants (cooked) contain	140
Gooseberries (raw) contain	40
Gooseberries (cooked) contain	28

A certain amount of nutrients pass into the cooking water when fruit is cooked, e.g., in stewed fruit and fruit pies. However, the 'juice' is eaten with the fruit so this is of no great importance. Prolonged soaking or washing of fruit should be avoided.

EFFECT OF COOKING UTENSILS ON FOOD

The materials used in the manufacture of saucepans, casseroles and earthenware vessels for food preparation, have little or no effect on the nutritive value of the food.

Aluminium utensils are generally very resistant to corrosion by foods and do not accelerate the destruction of vitamins or other nutrients during cooking. Acid fruits, and vegetables to which bicarbonate of soda has been added, have a slightly corrosive effect but aluminium is too insoluble to be absorbed by the body.

Hollow-ware enamels are made up of several materials and can be 'hard' or 'soft' according to their silica content. Hollow-ware articles made with seams, e.g., water cans, jugs, buckets, are usually coated with the 'soft' cheap enamel which deteriorates readily at the seams. The organic acids in foods, especially tartaric acid, will dissolve the outer glaze and so enable harmful substances, such as antimony salts, to be taken up by the food. The same applies to cheap enamels which are chipped. In 'hard' enamels, however, there is no danger as the enamel is more resistant and a chip would only expose the iron below the glaze. In this case small amounts of iron may be absorbed beneficially.

Lead may be present in cheap enamels and lead glazes are occasionally used for casseroles and earthenware articles. Acid liquids, especially when hot, may dissolve a considerable amount of lead if left in such containers for some time. Acid liquids, such as lemonade, should not, therefore, be allowed to stand for any length of time in cheap enamel pans or those with lead glazes.

Non-stick utensils coated with polytetrafluoroethylene resin remain inert at normal cooking temperatures and are safe for conventional kitchen use. It is important to avoid scratching the lining or the special properties will be lost.

The use of *cast iron* pans can be beneficial in that small traces of iron may be consumed. However, their use may cause discoloration of foods in cooking as with the blackening of potatoes.

If *copper* is kept clean it is not readily attacked by foods. In contact with fruit juices, oxidation occurs and a dark film forms on the surface which can be dissolved by foods more easily than the copper. It is non-toxic, but traces of copper have a catalytic action on the oxidation and destruction of vitamin C. Copper pans, however, are usually lined with tin. Long cooking with acid solutions may cause this lining to be dissolved, e.g., in tomato purée, so exposing the copper.

EFFECT OF COOKING ON MINERAL SUBSTANCES

Calcium. Cooking may effect the calcium in foods in two ways, but neither is of great importance. In milk, for example, heat may cause a slight reduction in the availability of calcium to the body, whereas in cereals calcium may become more available.

An indirect effect of cooking on the amount of calcium in foods is that of the calcium in hard cooking water. For example, if vegetables are boiled in hard water their total calcium content may increase by nearly a quarter; conversely, vegetables boiled in soft water will lose calcium during cooking.

Iron. A way in which iron may be lost during cooking is by discarding the resulting juices after cooking meat.

Sodium. Salt (sodium chloride) may be lost from foods when they are boiled. This is of little nutritional significance, since salt is always added during cooking.

Meals

A meal can be arbitrarily defined as an amount of food eaten during a single space of time and providing 200 kcal or more. This definition includes a great deal more than is generally accepted as the meaning of the word 'meal', which, in its popular sense, is usually restricted to the consumption of cooked and hot food by a person or persons sitting down.

NUMBER OF MEALS A DAY

People may eat three, four, five or six meals a day. Conditions of work and the time taken in travelling to and from work will determine the most convenient arrangement. Although the amounts of nutrients in different meals may vary, the total intake of each nutrient during the day must meet individual needs if the day's food is to be fully adequate for health.

There is some evidence that the number of meals in a day (and consequently the amount of food eaten at one time) influences the pattern of utilization of food by the body.

CALCULATION OF THE COMPOSITION OF PREPARED DISHES

In Appendix A, the composition of foodstuffs is given in terms of nutrients. The determination of the nutritional value of dishes made from several ingredients is usually a matter of arithmetic based on the figures given there. To illustrate this, the calculation of the nutritional value of a steak and kidney pie is shown in Table 4 (page 63).

CALCULATION OF THE COMPOSITION OF MEALS

It is quite common to find, particularly in canteens, two types of meals being served; one the sandwich-type, the other a cooked meal. The first, for example, may consist of two 'cheese rolls' and a cup of tea. Where little is known of the principles of nutrition this might not be considered to be a meal at all. The second could consist of roast lamb, cabbage and potato, followed by apple pie and cream.

The nutritional value of two such meals has been calculated in Table 5 on page 64 from the figures given in Appendix A.

These calculations show that *Meal 1*, which might be dismissed as a mere 'snack', is, in some ways, of higher nutritional value than the hot *Meal 2*. Thus it provides about the same amount of protein, nearly four times as much calcium and two and a half times as much vitamin A, but less energy and some other nutrients.

The vitamin C content of the second meal is markedly superior to the first. If the cheese roll had included watercress or tomato, or had been accompanied by an orange, it would have been in some ways nutritionally a better meal than the meat, vegetables and pudding and its lower energy value might have been an advantage.

This need not, of course, always be the case when 'packed' meals or snacks are compared with 'cooked' meals. Whether it is or not depends on the quantities and the nutritional composition of the items chosen for each meal.

The '*Oslo Breakfast*' which was introduced into the schools of Norway in the late 1920s is an illustration of a practical and *economical* sandwich meal for Norwegians with a *high nutritional value*. It consisted of milk with sandwiches made of rye bread, vitaminized margarine, whey cheese, cod liver paste, and a raw carrot, apple or orange according to the time of year.

WASTE

In studying the composition of meals, the information needed is the amount of each nutrient actually eaten. When the nutritional value of the meals, and hence of the total diet, of any individual has been calculated, it is possible to compare the values with the intakes recommended for health. It is important to remember, however, that it is not possible to calculate the nutritional value of a diet directly from the total amounts of foods bought from the shop, or from the amounts used in the kitchen. There is always a proportion of waste for which allowance must be made, for example:

(1) potato peelings, bacon rind, bones from meat, crusts cut off bread, outer leaves of cabbage, etc.;
(2) fat lost on pans, batter left in mixing bowls, etc.;
(3) scraps left on plates, bread, etc., wasted at table;
(4) food fed to domestic pets, birds and animals.

Before calculating the nutritional adequacy of any diets allowance must be made for wastage (unless it is possible to measure the amounts of edible food actually eaten). The average loss of edible material often assumed for wastage in cooking and from plates is 10 per cent, but, of course, the figure varies according to circumstances. When using the food tables in Appendix A which refer only to 'edible portion', a further deduction may be necessary for skins, bones, stones, outer leaves, shells, etc., in order to arrive at the edible weight of food if only the 'as purchased' weight is known. Average figures for this loss of inedible material are given in the first column of the Tables (see also page 45).

EATING BETWEEN MEALS

There seems to be no important nutritional argument for or against eating small quantities of food between meals, provided that the day's total consumption of nutrients is not prejudiced. But if children eat sweets (which are largely composed of sugar and provide no other nutrient than carbohydrate) between meals, so that they have no appetite for vegetables or for meat at dinner later, the consumption of sweets may then have reduced the amount

TABLE 4

Nutrients in Steak and Kidney Pie

Food	Weight	Energy value	Protein	Fat	Carbohydrate	Calcium	Iron	Vitamin A (retinol equivalents)	Vitamin D	Thiamine	Riboflavine	Nicotinic acid equivalents (f)
	g	kcal	g	g	g	mg	mg	µg	µg	mg	mg	mg
Beef, stewing raw	425	901	72·2	68·0	0	42	17·0	0	0	0·18(c)	0·76(e)	31·4(e)
Kidney, raw	200	210	33·8	8·4	0	28	26·8	600	0	0·36(c)	3·60(e)	20·0(e)
Flour	190	661	19·0	1·7	152·0	276	3·6	0	0	0·45(d)	0·08	5·3
Margarine	65	500	0·1	55·4	0	3	0·2	585(b)	5·20(b)	0	0	0
Lard	65	581	0	64·5	0	0	0	0	0	0	0	0
Water	195											
Whole pie	940(a)	2,853	125·1	198·0	152·0	349	47·6	1,185	5·20	0·99	4·44	56·7
Composition per 100 g	100	304	13·3	21·1	16·2	37	5·1	126	0·55	0·11	0·47	6·0
Composition per oz	1	86	3·8	6·0	4·6	10	1·4	36	0·16	0·03	0·13	1·7

(a) The total weight will not be the same as the sum of ingredients owing to the loss of moisture on cooking.

(b) Margarine for home consumption contains vitamins A and D; these vitamins would not necessarily be present in a bought pie.

(c) 40 per cent deducted to allow for loss in cooking.

(d) 15 per cent deducted to allow for loss in cooking.

(e) 10 per cent deducted to allow for loss in cooking.

(f) Available nicotinic acid $+\frac{\text{tryptophan}}{60}$

Table 5

Meal 1

Food	Weight	Energy value	Protein	Fat	Carbohydrate	Calcium	Iron	Vitamin A (retinol equivalents)	Vitamin D	Thiamine	Riboflavine	Nicotinic acid equivalents(b)	Vitamin C
	oz	kcal	g	g	g	mg	mg	μg	μg	mg	mg	mg	mg
Rolls(a)	3·5	252	8·4	1·8	54·2	98	1·8	0	0	0·18	0	2·4	0
Butter	0·3	63	0	7·0	0	1	0	85	0·11	0	0	0	0
Cheese	2·0	234	14·4	19·6	0	460	0·4	238	0·20	0·02	0·28	3·0	0
Tea	0·1	0	0	0	0	0	0	0	0	0	0·03	0·2	0
Milk (summer)	1·0	19	0·9	1·1	1·4	34	0	12	0·01	0·01	0·04	0·3	0(d)
Total meal		568	23·7	29·5	55·6	593	2·2	335	0·32	0·21	0·35	5·9	0

Meal 2

Food	Weight	Energy value	Protein	Fat	Carbohydrate	Calcium	Iron	Vitamin A (retinol equivalents)	Vitamin D	Thiamine	Riboflavine	Nicotinic acid equivalents(b)	Vitamin C
	oz	kcal	g	g	g	mg	mg	μg	μg	mg	mg	mg	mg
Lamb, roast	2·7	219	19·2	15·7	0	3	3·2	0	0	0·08	0·19	7·6	0
Cabbage, boiled	3·0	6	0·6	0	1·2	48	0·3	42	0	0·03	0·03	0·3	18
Potato, boiled	4·0	92	1·6	0	22·4	4	0·4	0	0	0·08	0·04	1·2	4–16(c)
Apple pie	4·0	332	3·6	16·4	46·0	48	0·8	4	0	0·08	0·04	1·2	4
Cream, single	2·0	108	1·6	10·2	2·4	56	0	88	0·03	0·02	0·08	0·4	0(d)
Total meal		757	26·6	42·3	72·0	159	4·7	134	0·03	0·29	0·38	10·7	26–38

(a) Calculated as white bread.

(b) Available nicotinic acid $+ \frac{\text{tryptophan}}{60}$

(c) Vitamin C falls in storage.

(d) Less than 1 mg

of vitamin C or of protein which could have been obtained from the vegetables and the meat. If excessive, the practice can also be bad for the teeth. The cleansing action of raw apples makes them particularly suitable as snacks for children.

Eating high carbohydrate foods between meals can also lead to an undesirable increase in weight if the energy value of the *total daily food intake* then exceeds the energy used up.

WORKING BEFORE BREAKFAST

The efficiency of the muscles is lowest in the morning before the first meal of the day. It is, therefore, good nutritional practice to eat breakfast before starting work, particularly for children.

Planning Balanced Meals

MEALS are well balanced when they provide adequate amounts of proteins, minerals, vitamins and energy. The amounts of nutrients recommended daily for health for every type of individual are discussed on pages 42 to 44, and the figures given there show the results to aim at when a diet is being planned. Most foods contain several nutrients, therefore a great variety of foods, which are commonly eaten in the United Kingdom, can be combined to provide these specified amounts. The main sources of each nutrient have already been discussed. Food choice is strongly influenced by experience and custom, often in such a way that meals are nutritionally satisfactory as well as good to eat; nevertheless, to be sure that this is achieved a general plan should be followed.

Each main meal should contain:

(*a*) Some foods rich in *protein* (see pages 9–12). The most important are meat, poultry and fish, cheese, eggs, and milk, all of which provide animal protein; also vegetable protein foods, such as bread and flour, nuts, peas and beans.

(*b*) Plenty of *fruit and vegetables:* these are rich sources of some vitamins and minerals.

Sugary foods and foods containing a high proportion of starch or of fat, which are eaten primarily to provide *energy*, should be included in amounts which will satisfy appetite and maintain a steady body weight.

Within this general framework it is often necessary to consider the relative cost of different sources of nutrients.

YOUNG CHILDREN

For the first few months of their lives infants can live satisfactorily on their mother's milk. Although milk is a remarkably complete food, it is not perfect in every respect for a growing child. For example:

Cow's milk is deficient in vitamin C. Babies must be given orange juice or some other source of vitamin C, if milk is their main food.

Vitamin A and vitamin D are present in milk, but not in sufficient amounts for the child as it begins to grow; supplements, such as cod liver oil or capsules containing vitamins A and D, must therefore be given.

Milk is lacking in iron. When it is born, a child usually possesses sufficient iron stored in its liver for its needs for some months. It is, however, important not to delay too long before beginning to feed small amounts of other foods, such as egg yolk, in order to provide the infant with this nutrient.

Dried milk is easy to handle and a variety of proprietary products are available. Many manufacturers add vitamins and other nutrients, such as iron, to the milk powder and it is important to read the information on the label, which gives the amounts of nutrients which the milk will supply when reconstituted according to the instructions.

After the first few months, fluid and semi-fluid infant cereal foods, egg yolk, homogenized vegetables and fruit and finely divided meat are used to supplement cow's milk and the diet undergoes a gradual transition to solid food. By 9 months to one year, the infant is eating a mixed diet not very different from the remainder of the family. More details about feeding infants and young children will be found in the books recommended for supplementary reading on page 102.

SCHOOLCHILDREN

Three points are of great importance:

Schoolchildren are growing fast and therefore have great need for protein, calcium, vitamin A, vitamin C and vitamin D. The intakes recommended can be seen in the Table on page 42.

Schoolchildren are very active and therefore have, for their size, greater need for energy than adults. Children's big appetites almost always reflect a real nutritional need, not greediness.

Children need a large amount of nutrients, but because of their small size and correspondingly small stomachs, it is important that their *meals should not be too bulky*. Bread and, particularly, cake made with fat, sugar, milk and eggs are excellent as concentrated sources of energy. Cheese, meat, eggs, fruit and green vegetables are all important to supply children with the nutrients they need. Of all other foods milk is the best source for schoolchildren of protein, calcium and riboflavine.

School Meals

Under the Provision of Milk and Meals Regulations, 1969, made by the Secretary of State for Education and Science, school dinners should be provided which are suitable in all respects as the main meal of the day.

The nutritional standard of the school dinner is based on recommendations made in 1965* which are set out in Circular 3/66† issued by the Department of Education and Science to local education authorities. The total nutritional value per average meal should be 29 g protein, including approximately 18·5 g animal protein, and 32 g fat in all forms; and the meal should

* Report of the Departmental Working Party on the Nutritional Standard of the School Dinner HMSO 1965.

† Department of Education and Science: The Nutritional Standard of the School Dinner. Jan. 1966.

have an average energy value of 880 kcal. Special provision for the adjustment of these nutrients for different age groups is not thought necessary, as the variations in the size of the portion served to children of different ages and sex will automatically regulate the protein and calorie value of the meals served. Meals reaching these standards also provide suitable amounts of vitamins and minerals.

ADOLESCENTS

The nutrient needs of adolescents are higher in many respects than those of any other group. Healthy adolescents have very big appetites, and it is important that they should satisfy them with food of high nutritional value in the form of well balanced meals. The increase in obesity among schoolchildren is considerable, and this frequently continues into adult life. A knowledge of nutrition and its application at this time may easily benefit the health of young people for the rest of their lives.

ADULTS

The arrangement of meals in different occupations has already been discussed. It depends on the length of the working shift, whether the work is indoors or out-of-doors, and on many other conditions. In general, it seems best for the nutrients to be spaced out fairly evenly throughout the day. As physical activity decreases the energy value of the diet should be reduced. If this adjustment is not made, the energy from all food which is in excess of physiological needs will be stored in the body in the form of fat. Obesity is detrimental to health in many ways and, if allowed to progress, can lead to a reduction in the expectation of life.

OLD PEOPLE

Old people sometimes present special dietary problems because they may be arthritic, or of senile mentality, or have failing vision or difficulty in mastication. Because of this they are sometimes found to be on a very restricted diet. Their energy needs are lower than those of younger adults, and the problem is to give them meals which provide adequate amounts of all nutrients without excess energy. Moreover, some may need meals that require little or no cooking; and for these eggs, cheese, tinned meats or fish and milk are useful. Old people sometimes develop scurvy, because they are on a restricted diet. Prevention may be achieved by adhering to a rule of eating an orange *at least* twice weekly; this has the virtue of simplicity. If, however, the old person does not care for oranges, tomatoes or other suitable fresh or even canned fruits can be suggested, though rather more should be eaten. When the old person is able to cope with the necessary preparation, meat, fish and offal are greatly preferable to such foods as cake, sweets and sugary foods which are sources of energy, but do not make many other useful contributions to the diet.

ATHLETES

Provided that an adequate diet is given, there is no certain way of improving athletic performance by means of food. The individual undergoing heavy physical exercise will have a very greatly increased need for energy, but so long as this is provided, a well balanced diet will supply adequate nutrients to meet the recommended intakes.

FOOD ALLERGIES

The principles set out in this book hold, in general, for all normal individuals. There are, however, a few people who possess personal idiosyncrasies which cause reactions to certain foods, for example, shell-fish or strawberries. Such allergies usually present a medical rather than a nutritional problem.

MEASUREMENT OF FOOD CONSUMPTION

It is important not only that all nutrients needed should be present in the foods eaten, but also that they should be present in the amounts required by different people.

Thus, in trying to find out whether a particular diet is adequate three things must be known:

(1) What foods were eaten?

(2) How much of each food was eaten?

(3) What kind of people ate the foods? Were they men, women, adolescents, or children, and were they very active or sedentary? Were any of the women pregnant or nursing a baby?

Two important ways of finding out about diets involve answering one or other of the following questions:

(1) How much food was bought for example, by a family, during one week, and how many people ate it? If the amount of food bought is recorded, it is important to know how much of it is eaten, how much goes into or out of the store-cupboard, and how much is wasted in preparing meals and on the plate.

(2) What weights of foods were eaten by an individual at each separate meal for, say, one week? This is probably the most precise method of assessing the value of a diet; each item of food must be weighed and recorded and any plate waste deducted.

For meals served by canteens or restaurants it is, of course, possible to weigh all the ingredients of a number of meals when ready for serving. An estimate of the amounts of nutrients wasted in preparation can be obtained by comparing the calculated nutritional value of the meals served with the calculated nutritional value of the supplies of food entering the kitchen (See also page 62).

ASSESSMENT OF THE ADEQUACY OF DIETS

An understanding of nutrition is important for the appreciation of diets found in practise. An example is given overleaf.

Menu for One Day for Women doing Normal Work

Breakfast	Cornflakes (½ oz) Milk (4 oz) Sugar (¼ oz)	Boiled egg (2 oz)	Toast (2 oz) Butter (½ oz) Marmalade (½ oz)	2 cups of tea* Milk (2 oz) Sugar (½ oz)
Snack .	One cup of coffee*	Milk (2 oz) Sugar (¼ oz)		
Lunch .	Tomato soup (6 oz) Cheese salad	Cheese (2 oz) Lettuce (1 oz) Tomato (2½ oz) Beetroot (1½ oz) Watercress (½ oz)	Bread (2 oz) Butter (½ oz) Fruit yoghurt (5 oz)	One cup of coffee* Milk (2 oz) Sugar (¼ oz)
Snack .	Two cups of tea* Plain biscuit (½ oz)	Milk (2 oz) Sugar (½ oz)		
Supper .	Roast chicken (3 oz) Peas (3 oz) Brussels sprouts (3 oz) Roast potatoes (4 oz)		Canned peaches (4 oz) Single cream (2 oz)	

* The amount of tea or coffee used varies considerably. These arbitrary figures have been used per cup: tea 1/6 oz, coffee 1/10 oz.

The nutrients obtained from this menu are shown in the Table on p. 70. These can be compared with the figures on page 42, which show the amounts recommended for health, giving the comparison shown in Table 6.

TABLE 6

Nutrient Intake		Amounts recommended for Health
Energy	2224 kcal	Most women need 2,200 kcal per day so that the amount eaten is about the amount needed.
Protein	89·8 g	Since women need approximately 55 g protein per day, the amount obtained is more than adequate.
Calcium	1,461 mg	This is plenty since approximately 500 mg is recommended.
Iron	13·1 mg	This is enough since approximately 12 mg is recommended.
Vitamin A (retinol equivalents)	1,367 μg	This is enough since approximately 750 μg is recommended.
Vitamin D	1·61 μg	This amount is less than the recommended 2·5 μg but can be considered sufficient. No dietary source may be necessary for those adequately exposed to sunlight.
Thiamine	1·14 mg	This is sufficient since approximately 0·9 mg is recommended.
Riboflavine	2·07 mg	This is sufficient since approximately 1·3 mg is recommended.
Nicotinic acid equivalents	32·9 mg	This is fully sufficient since approximately 15 mg is recommended.
Vitamin C	93 mg	This quantity exceeds the recommended amount of 30 mg.

TABLE 7

Diet for Women doing Normal Work (See page 69)

Meal	Energy value	Protein	Fat	Carbohydrate	Calcium	Iron	Vitamin A (retinol equivalents)	Vitamin D	Thiamine	Riboflavine	Nicotinic acid equivalents	Vitamin C
	kcal	g	g	g	mg	mg	µg	µg	mg	mg	mg	mg
Breakfast . .	627	18·1	26·3	83·9	300	2·7	378	1·09	0·30	0·59	6·5	2
Snack . . .	70	1·9	2·2	11·2	72	0·1	22	0·02	0·02	0·08	1·9	0
Lunch . .	811	30·2	42·4	83·7	883	3·1	710	0·42	0·33	0·75	8·2	41
Snack . . .	155	2·9	4·0	28·3	86	0·4	22	0·02	0·05	0·19	1·5	0
Supper . .	561	36·7	17·7	67·3	120	6·8	235	0·06	0·44	0·46	14·8	50
Total day's nutrients	2,224	89·8	92·6	274·4	1,461	13·1	1,367	1·61	1·14	2·07	32·9	93

Methods of Teaching Nutrition

THE approach which is most useful in teaching nutrition depends, of course, on the members of the class, their previous knowledge of allied subjects, their age and aptitude, as well as on the time that can be devoted to the subject.

Three broad methods have been used; it is for the teacher to decide which is most appropriate for his or her purpose. *First*, nutrition can be taught in terms of the chemical nature of nutrients. If this method is used, the audience should preferably have some knowledge of a relevant scientific discipline and of cooking and catering; further, they must be able to devote a fair amount of time to the course. This Manual has been prepared on these lines, and could well form the basis of such a course. A suggested outline is given in Appendix B.

The *second* approach is based on the functions of foods, is simpler to use, and very little background knowledge is necessary. It is known as the Three Food Groups, i.e., body-building, protective, and energy-giving foods. This method was largely developed during World War II, when rationing was in force; it was an effective way of expressing food requirements in quantitative terms against a background of food control, but it is less easy to express in these terms in present-day conditions.

Body-building foods are considered to be those which contain the nutrients for building and maintaining the skeleton—calcium; the muscles—protein; and the blood system—iron. Protective foods are those which contain vitamins. Energy foods are those which are good sources of fat and carbohydrate and, to a certain extent, protein.

These two methods can be linked together in the following way, and teaching can also be based on this:

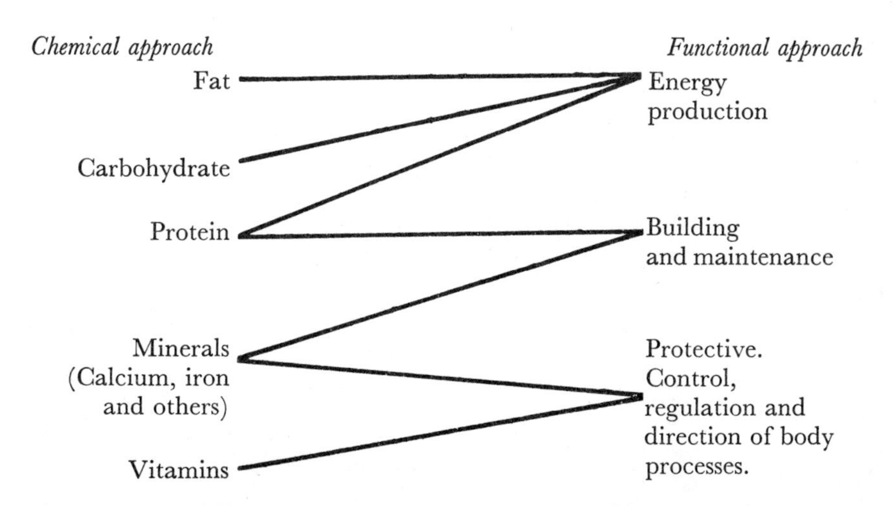

The *third* approach is in terms of foods. This method has been used for simple nutrition teaching in the United States of America, Canada and other countries; it is based on foods grouped according to their contribution of nutrients to the diet and expressed quantitatively in the number of portions of each group of foods which should be taken daily. Further details of this approach can be obtained from American and Canadian text-books.

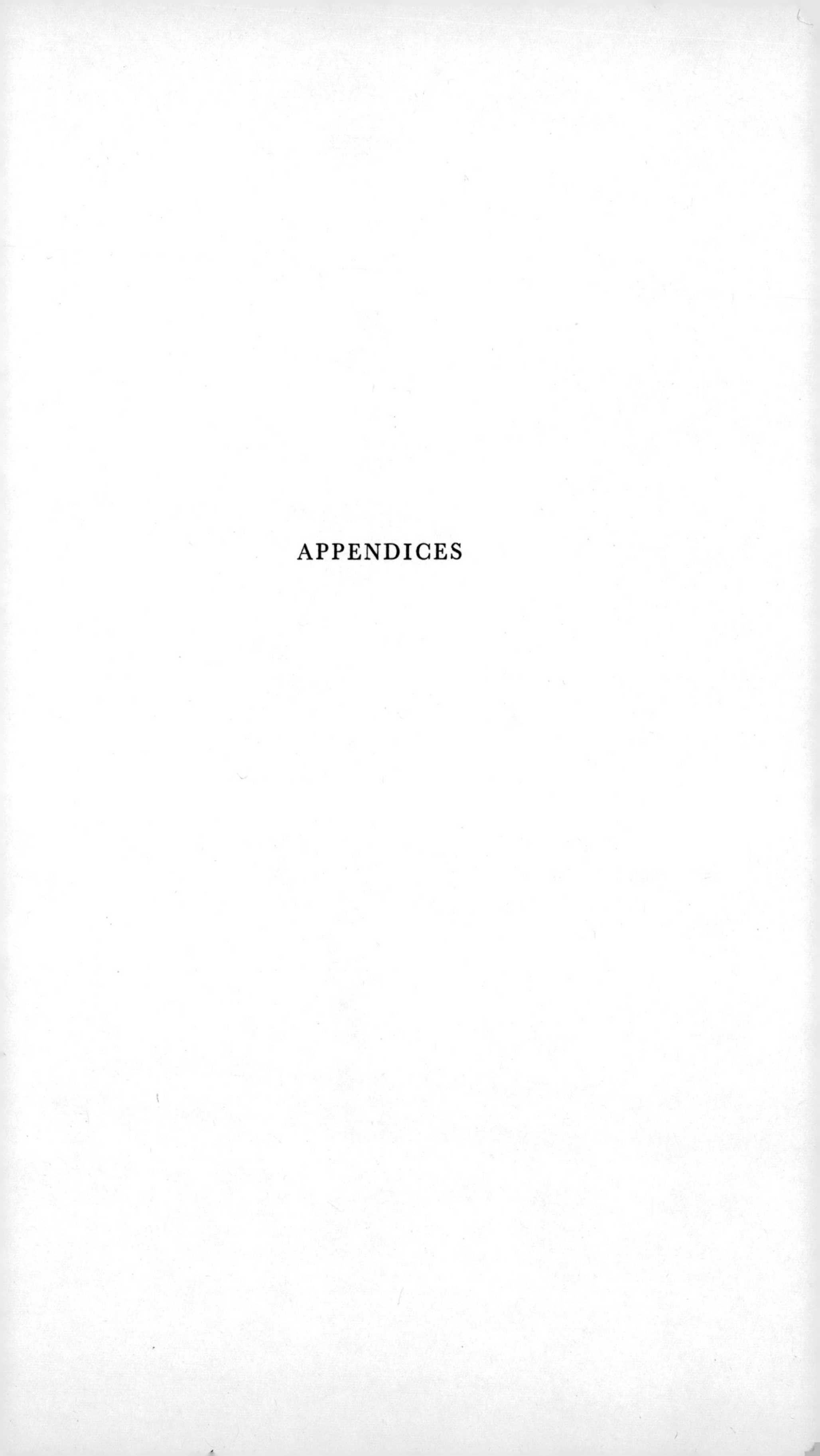

APPENDICES

Appendix A

COMPOSITION OF FOOD

The composition of food is given in three tables:

Table 1: Composition per 100 g

Table 2: Composition per ounce

Table 3: Composition per 100 kcal

The figures are for the *raw edible portion of the food unless otherwise stated.* The tables are based chiefly on 'The Composition of Foods' by R. A. McCance and E. M. Widdowson.

Two of the vitamins are given in the tables in the form of equivalents; these are vitamin A (as retinol equivalents, see p. 24, and nicotinic acid equivalents (see p. 29). In the following tables, total nicotinic acid refers to the content of nicotinic acid alone; nicotinic acid equivalents include the contribution from tryptophan. The two vitamins are thus expressed in the same form as in the Recommended Intakes of Nutrients for the U.K. of the Department of Health and Social Security (see p. 42).

In Tables 1 and 2 the energy value for the foods is given in kilojoules (kJ) as well as kilocalories; kilojoules are calculated from kilocalories using the relationship 1 kcal=4·19 kJ.

TABLE 1

Composition of foods per 100 g

No.	Food	Inedible waste	Energy value		Protein	Fat	Carbohydrate (as monosaccharide)
		%	kcal	kJ	g	g	g
	Milk						
1	Cream, double	0	449	1,881	1·8	48·0	2·6
2	Cream, single	0	189	792	2·8	18·0	4·2
3	Milk, liquid, whole	0	65	272	3·3	3·8	4·8
4	Milk, condensed, whole, sweetened	0	322	1,349	8·2	9·2	55·1
5	Milk, whole, evaporated	0	166	696	8·5	9·2	12·8
6	Milk, dried, whole	0	492	2,061	26·6	27·7	37·6
7	Milk, dried, half-cream	0	425	1,781	31·5	15·0	43·8
8	Milk, dried, skimmed	0	329	1,379	37·2	0·5	46·9
9	Yoghurt, natural	0	57	239	3·6	2·6	5·2
10	Yoghurt, fruit	0	79	331	3·6	1·8	13·0
	Cheese						
11	Cheese, Cheddar	0	412	1,726	25·4	34·5	0
12	Cheese, cottage	0	115	482	15·3	4·0	4·5
	Meat						
13	Bacon, average	13	476	1,994	11·0	48·0	0
14	Beef, average	17	313	1,311	14·8	28·2	0
15	Beef, corned	0	224	939	22·3	15·0	0
16	Beef, stewing steak, raw	0	212	888	17·0	16·0	0
17	Beef, stewing steak, cooked	0	242	1,014	29·0	14·0	0
18	Chicken, raw	31	144	603	20·8	6·7	0
19	Chicken, roast	—	184	771	29·6	7·3	0
20	Ham, cooked	0	422	1,768	16·3	39·6	0
21	Kidney, average	0	105	440	16·9	4·2	0
22	Lamb, average, raw	17	331	1,387	13·0	31·0	0
23	Lamb, roast	—	284	1,190	25·0	20·4	0
24	Liver, average, raw	0	139	582	16·5	8·1	0
25	Liver, fried	0	276	1,156	29·5	15·9	4·0
26	Luncheon meat	0	325	1,362	11·4	29·0	5·0
27	Pork, average	15	408	1,710	12·0	40·0	0
28	Pork chop, grilled	40	527	2,208	18·6	50·3	0
29	Sausage, pork	0	369	1,546	10·4	30·9	13·3
30	Steak and kidney pie, cooked	0	304	1,274	13·3	21·1	16·2
31	Tripe	0	60	251	11·6	1·0	0
	Fish						
32	Cod, haddock, white fish	40	69	289	16·0	0·5	0
33	Cod, fried in batter	0	199	834	19·6	10·3	7·5

TABLE 1—*contd.*

Composition per 100 *g*

No.	Calcium	Iron	Vitamin A (retinol equivalents)	Vitamin D	Thiamine	Riboflavine	Nicotinic acid		Vitamin C
							Total	Equivalents	
	mg	mg	μg	μg	mg	mg	mg	mg	mg
1	65	0	420	0·28	0·02	0·08	0	0·4	0
2	100	0·1	155	0·10	0·03	0·13	0·1	0·8	1
3	120	0·1	44 (a) 37 (b)	0·05 (a) 0·01 (b)	0·04	0·15	0·1	0·9	1(e)
4	290	0·2	112	0·12	0·10	0·40	0·2	2·0	3
5	290	0·2	112	0·12	0·06	0·37	0·2	2·0	2
6	813	0·7	246	0·30 (c) 8·82 (d)	0·31	1·10	0·7	6·9	11
7	940	0·8	143	0·18 (c) 8·82 (d)	0·36	1·35	1·0	8·2	10
8	1,277	1·1	4	0	0·30	1·73	1·1	9·7	10
9	140	0·1	39	0·02	0·05	0·19	0·1	0·9	0
10	140	0·1	22	0·02	0·05	0·19	0·1	0·9	0
11	810	0·6	420	0·35	0·04	0·50	0·1	5·2	0
12	80	0·4	27	0·02	0·03	0·27	0·1	3·2	0
13	10	1·0	0	0	0·40	0·15	1·5	4·0	0
14	10	4·0	0	0	0·07	0·20	5·0	7·8	0
15	13	9·8	0	0	0	0·20	3·5	7·7	0
16	10	4·0	0	0	0·07	0·20	5·0	8·2	0
17	8	5·0	0	0	0·05	0·22	5·0	10·4	0
18	11	1·5	0	0	0·04	0·17	5·9	9·5	0
19	15	2·6	0	0	0·04	0·14	4·9	10·0	0
20	13	2·5	0	0	0·50	0·20	3·5	7·2	0
21	14	13·4	300	0	0·30	2·00	7·0	11·1	12
22	10	2·0	0	0	0·15	0·25	5·0	7·7	0
23	4	4·3	0	0	0·10	0·25	4·5	9·8	0
24	8	13·9	6,000	0·75	0·30	3·00	13·0	17·1	30
25	9	20·7	6,000	0·75	0·30	3·50	15·0	22·4	20
26	18	1·1	0	0	0·40	0·20	3·5	6·1	0
27	10	1·0	0	0	1·00	0·20	5·0	7·7	0
28	8	2·4	0	0	0·80	0·20	5·0	9·2	0
29	15	2·5	0	0	0·17	0·07	1·6	3·9	0
30	37	5·1	126	0·55	0·11	0·47	4·1	6·0	0
31	70	0·7	10	0	0·18	0·10	3·5	5·7	0
32	25	1·0	0	0	0·06	0·10	3·0	6·0	0
33	80	0·5	0	0	0·04	0·10	3·0	6·7	0

(a) Summer value (b) Winter value. (c) natural value. (d) with fortification.
(e) Less than 1 mg.

TABLE 1—*contd.*

Composition per 100 *g*

No.	Food	Inedible waste	Energy value		Protein	Fat	Carbohydrate (as monosaccharide)
		%	kcal	kJ	g	g	g
	Fish cont.:						
34	Fish fingers	0	192	804	13·4	6·8	20·7
35	Herring	37	190	796	16·0	14·1	0
36	Kipper	40	220	922	19·0	16·0	0
37	Salmon, canned	2	133	557	19·7	6·0	0
38	Sardines, canned in oil	0	285	1,194	20·4	22·6	0
	Eggs						
39	Eggs, fresh	12	158	662	11·9	12·3	0
	Fats						
40	Butter	0	745	3,122	0·5	82·5	0
41	Lard, cooking fat dripping	0	894	3,746	0	99·3	0
42	Margarine	0	769	3,222	0·2	85·3	0
43	Oils, cooking and salad	0	899	3,767	0	99·9	0
	Preserves etc.						
44	Chocolate, milk	0	578	2,422	8·7	37·6	54·5
45	Honey	0	288	1,207	0·4	0	76·4
46	Jam	0	262	1,098	0·5	0	69·2
47	Ice cream, vanilla	0	192	805	4·1	11·3	19·8
48	Marmalade	0	261	1,094	0·1	0	69·5
49	Sugar, white	0	394	1,651	0	0	105·0
50	Syrup	0	297	1,244	0·3	0	79·0
	Vegetables						
51	Beans canned in tomato sauce	0	92	385	6·0	0·4	17·3
52	Beans, broad	75	69	289	7·2	0·5	9·5
53	Beans, haricot	0	256	1,073	21·4	0	45·5
54	Beans, runner	14	15	63	1·1	0	2·9
55	Beetroot, boiled	20	44	184	1·8	0	9·9
56	Brussels sprouts, raw	25	32	134	3·6	0	4·6
57	Brussels sprouts, boiled	0	16	67	2·4	0	1·7
58	Cabbage, raw	30	28	117	1·5	0	5·8
59	Cabbage, boiled	0	8	34	0·8	0	1·3
60	Carrots, old	4	23	96	0·7	0	5·4
61	Cauliflower	30	24	101	3·4	0	2·8
62	Celery	27	8	34	0·9	0	1·3
63	Lentils, dry	0	295	1,236	23·8	0	53·2
64	Lettuce	20	11	46	1·1	0	1·8
65	Mushrooms	25	7	29	1·8	0	0
66	Onions	3	23	96	0·9	0	5·2
67	Parsnips	26	49	205	1·7	0	11·3
68	Peas, fresh raw or quick frozen	63	63	264	5·8	0	10·6

TABLE 1—*contd.*

Composition per 100 g

No.	Calcium	Iron	Vitamin A (retinol equivalents)	Vitamin D	Thiamine	Riboflavine	Nicotinic acid Total	Nicotinic acid Equivalents	Vitamin C
	mg	mg	µg	µg	mg	mg	mg	mg	mg
34	50	1·4	0	0	0·12	0·16	1·8	3·9	0
35	100	1·5	45	22·25	0·03	0·30	3·5	6·4	0
36	120	2·0	45	22·25	0	0·30	3·5	6·9	0
37	66	1·3	90	12·50	0·03	0·10	7·0	10·6	0
38	409	4·0	30	7·50	0	0·20	5·0	8·6	0
39	56	2·5	300	1·50	0·10	0·35	0·1	3·0	0
40	15	0·2	995	1·25	0	0	0	0·1	0
41	0	0	0	0	0	0	0	0	0
42	4	0·3	900 (e)	8·00	0	0	0	0·1	0
43	0	0	0	0	0	0	0	0	0
44	246	1·7	6·6	0	0·03	0·35	1·0	2·5	0
45	5	0·4	0	0	0	0·05	0·2	0·2	0
46	18	1·2	2	0	0	0	0	0	10
47	137	0·3	1	0	0·05	0·20	0·1	1·1	1
48	35	0·6	8	0	0	0	0	0	10
49	1	0	0	0	0	0	0	0	0
50	26	1·4	0	0	0	0	0	0	0
51	62	2·1	50	0	0·06	0·04	0·5	1·5	3
52	30	1·1	22	0	0·28	0·05	4·0	5·0	30
53	180	6·7	0	0	0·45	0·13	2·5	6·1	0
54	33	0·7	50	0	0·05	0·10	0·9	1·2	20
55	30	0·7	0	0	0·02	0·04	0·1	0·4	5
56	29	0·7	67	0	0·10	0·16	0·7	1·4	100
57	27	0·6	67	0	0·06	0·10	0·4	0·9	35
58	65	1·0	50	0	0·06	0·05	0·2	0·5	60
59	58	0·5	50	0	0·03	0·03	0·2	0·3	20
60	48	0·6	2,000	0	0·06	0·05	0·6	0·7	6
61	18	0·6	5	0	0·10	0·10	0·6	1·4	70
62	52	0·6	0	0	0·03	0·03	0·3	0·5	7
63	39	7·6	6	0	0·50	0·25	2·5	6·3	0
64	26	0·7	167	0	0·07	0·08	0·3	0·4	15
65	3	1·0	0	0	0·10	0·40	4·0	4·5	3
66	31	0·3	0	0	0·03	0·05	0·2	0·4	10
67	55	0·6	0	0	0·10	0·09	1·0	1·3	15
68	15	1·9	50	0	0·32	0·15	2·5	3·5	25

(e) some margarines contain carotene.

TABLE 1—*contd.*

Composition per 100 g

No.	Food	Inedible waste	Energy value		Protein	Fat	Carbo-hydrate (as mono-saccharide)
		%	kcal	kJ	g	g	g
	Vegetables cont.:						
69	Peas, fresh, boiled or quick frozen boiled .	0	49	205	5·0	0	7·7
70	Peas, canned, processed . .	0	96	402	7·2	0	18·0
71	Peppers, green .	18	21	88	1·2	0·2	3·7
72	Potatoes, raw .	27 (f) 14 (g)	76	318	2·1	0	18·0
73	Potatoes, boiled .	0	79	331	1·4	0	19·7
74	Potato chips, fried .	0	236	989	3·8	9·0	37·3
75	Potatoes, roast .	0	123	515	2·8	1·0	27·3
76	Spinach . .	25	21	88	2·7	0	2·8
77	Sweet corn, canned	0	95	398	2·6	0·8	20·5
78	Tomatoes, fresh .	0	14	59	0·9	0	2·8
79	Turnips . .	16	17	71	0·8	0	3·8
80	Watercress . .	23	14	59	2·9	0	0·7
	Fruit						
81	Apple . . .	21	46	193	0·3	0	12·0
82	Apricots, canned .	0	106	444	0·5	0	27·7
83	Apricots, dried .	0	182	763	4·8	0	43·4
84	Bananas . .	40	76	318	1·1	0	19·2
85	Black currants .	2	28	117	0·9	0	6·6
86	Cherries . .	15	46	193	0·6	0	11·8
87	Dates . . .	14	248	1,039	2·0	0	63·9
88	Figs, dried . .	0	213	892	3·6	0	52·9
89	Gooseberries. .	1	27	113	0·9	0	6·3
90	Grapefruit . .	50	22	92	0·6	0	5·3
91	Lemons . .	64	7	29	0·3	0	1·6
92	Melon . . .	41	23	96	0·8	0	5·2
93	Oranges . .	25	35	147	0·8	0	8·5
94	Orange juice, canned unconcentrated .	0	47	197	0·8	0	11·7
95	Peaches, fresh .	13	37	155	0·6	0	9·1
96	Peaches, canned .	0	88	369	0·4	0	22·9
97	Pears, fresh . .	25	41	172	0·3	0	10·6
98	Pineapple, canned .	0	76	318	0·3	0	20·0
99	Plums . . .	8	32	134	0·6	0	7·9
100	Prunes. . .	17	161	675	2·4	0	40·3
101	Raspberries . .	0	25	105	0·9	0	5·6
102	Rhubarb . .	33	6	25	0·6	0	1·0
103	Strawberries . .	3	26	109	0·6	0	6·2
104	Sultanas . .	0	249	1,043	1·7	0	64·7
	Nuts						
105	Almonds . .	63	580	2,430	20·5	53·5	4·3
106	Coconut, desiccated	0	608	2,548	6·6	62·0	6·4
107	Peanuts, roasted .	0	586	2,455	28·1	49·0	8·6

(f) refers to old potatoes. (g) refers to new potatoes.

TABLE 1—*contd.*

composition per 100 *g*

No.	Calcium	Iron	Vitamin A (retinol equivalents)	Vitamin D	Thiamine	Riboflavine	Nicotinic acid Total	Nicotinic acid Equivalents	Vitamin C
	mg	mg	µg	µg	mg	mg	mg	mg	mg
69	13	1·2	50	0	0·25	0·11	1·5	2·3	15
70	29	1·1	67	0	0·06	0·04	0·5	1·6	2
71	9	0·7	42	0	0·08	0·08	0·5	0·7	128
72	8	0·7	0	0	0·11	0·04	1·2	1·8	8–30 (h)
73	4	0·5	0	0	0·08	0·03	0·8	1·2	4–15 (h)
74	14	1·4	0	0	0·10	0·04	1·2	2·2	6–20 (h)
75	10	1·0	0	0	0·10	0·04	1·2	2·0	6–23 (h)
76	70	3·2	1,000	0	0·12	0·20	0·6	1·3	60
77	5	0·5	35	0	0·03	0·05	0·9	0·3	4
78	13	0·4	117	0	0·06	0·04	0·6	0·7	20
79	59	0·4	0	0	0·04	0·05	0·6	0·8	25
80	222	1·6	500	0	0·10	0·16	0·6	2·0	60
81	4	0·3	5	0	0·04	0·02	0·1	0·1	5
82	12	0·7	166	0	0·02	0·01	0·3	0·3	5
83	92	4·1	600	0	0	0·20	3·0	3·4	0
84	7	0·4	33	0	0·04	0·07	0·6	0·8	10
85	60	1·3	33	0	0·03	0·06	0·3	0·3	200
86	18	0·4	20	0	0·05	0·06	0·3	0·4	5
87	68	1·6	10	0	0·07	0·04	2·0	2·3	0
88	284	4·2	8	0	0·10	0·13	1·7	2·2	0
89	22	0·4	30	0	0·04	0·03	0·3	0·4	40
90	17	0·3	0	0	0·05	0·02	0·2	0·3	40
91	8	0·1	0	0	0·02	0	0·1	0·1	50
92	16	0·4	160	0	0·05	0·03	0·5	0·5	25
93	41	0·3	8	0	0·10	0·03	0·2	0·3	50
94	10	0·4	8	0	0·07	0·02	0·2	0·2	40
95	5	0·4	83	0	0·02	0·05	1·0	1·1	8
96	3·5	1·9	41	0	0·01	0·02	0·6	0·6	4
97	8	0·2	2	0	0·03	0·03	0·2	0·3	3
98	13	1·7	7	0	0·05	0·02	0·2	0·3	8
99	12	0·3	37	0	0·05	0·03	0·5	0·6	3
100	38	2·9	160	0	0·10	0·20	1·5	1·7	0
101	41	1·2	13	0	0·02	0·03	0·4	0·5	25
102	103	0·4	10	0	0·01	0·07	0·3	0·3	10
103	22	0·7	5	0	0·02	0·03	0·4	0·5	60
104	52	1·8	0	0	0·10	0·30	0·5	0·6	0
105	247	4·2	0	0	0·32	0·25	2·0	4·9	0
106	22	3·6	0	0	0·06	0·04	0·6	1·8	0
107	61	2·0	0	0	0·23	0·10	16·0	20·8	0

(h) vitamin C falls during storage.

TABLE 1—*contd.*

Composition per 100 *g*

No.	Food	Inedible waste	Energy value		Protein	Fat	Carbohydrate (as monosaccharide)
		%	kcal	kJ	g	g	g
	Cereals						
108	Barley, pearl, dry	0	360	1,508	7·7	1·7	83·6
109	Biscuits, chocolate	0	497	2,082	7·1	24·9	65·3
110	Biscuits, plain, semi-sweet	0	431	1,806	7·4	13·2	75·3
111	Biscuits, rich, sweet	0	496	2,078	5·6	22·3	72·7
112	Bread, brown	0	237	993	9·2	1·8	49·0
113	Bread, starch reduced	0	234	980	10·5	1·5	47·6
114	Bread, white	0	253	1,060	8·3	1·7	54·6
115	Bread, wholemeal	0	241	1,010	9·6	3·1	46·7
116	Cornflakes	0	365	1,529	7·5	0·5	88·0
117	Custard powder, instant pudding, cornflour	0	353	1,479	0·5	0·7	92·0
118	Crispbread, Ryvita	0	318	1,332	10·0	2·1	69
119	Flour, white	0	348	1,458	10·0	0·9	80·0
120	Oatmeal	0	400	1,676	12·1	8·7	72·8
121	Rice	0	359	1,504	6·2	1·0	86·8
122	Spaghetti	0	364	1,525	9·9	1·0	84·0
	Beverages						
123	Black currant juice	0	229	960	0·2	0	60·9
124	Chocolate, drinking	0	410	1,718	5·6	6·8	87·0
125	Cocoa powder	0	446	1,869	18·8	22·5	45·0
126	Coffee, ground	0	0	0	0	0	0
127	Coffee, instant	0	156	654	4·0	0·7	35·5
128	Tea, dry	0	0	0	0	0	0
	Alcoholic Beverages						
129	Beer, mild, draught	0	25	105	0·2	0	1·6
130	Spirits, 70% proof	0	222	930	0	0	0
131	Wine, red	0	67	281	0·2	0	0·3
	Puddings and Cakes etc.						
132	Apple pie	0	294	1,231	3·2	14·4	40·4
133	Buns, currant	0	328	1,374	7·8	8·5	58·6
134	Fruit cake, rich	0	368	1,542	4·6	15·9	55·0
135	Jam tarts	0	391	1,638	3·2	13·8	67·7
136	Plain cake, Madeira	0	430	1,802	7·1	24·0	49·7
137	Rice pudding	0	142	595	3·6	7·6	15·7
138	Soup, tomato, canned	0	67	281	0·9	3·1	9·4
139	Trifle	0	162	679	3·1	5·6	26·5

TABLE 1—*contd.*

composition per 100 g

No.	Calcium	Iron	Vitamin A (retinol equivalents)	Vitamin D	Thiamine	Riboflavine	Nicotinic acid Total	Nicotinic acid Equivalents	Vitamin C
	mg	mg	μg	μg	mg	mg	mg	mg	mg
108	10	0·7	0	0	0·12	0·08	2·5	2·2	0
109	131	1·5	0	0	0·11	0·04	1·1	2·0	0
110	126	1·8	0	0	0·17	0·06	1·3	2·0	0
111	92	1·3	0	0	0·12	0·04	1·0	1·5	0
112	92	2·5	0	0	0·28	0·07	3·2	2·6	0
113	100	1·3	79	0	0·18	0·03	1·5	2·7	0
114	100	1·8	0	0	0·18	0·02	1·4	2·3	0
115	28	3·0	0	0	0·24	0·09	2·6	1·9	0
116	5	1·1	0	0	0·60	1·07	7·0	6·4	0
117	15	1·4	0	0	0	0	0	0·1	0
118	86	3·3	0	0	0·37	0·24	1·4	1·3	0
119	145	1·9	0	0	0·28	0·04	1·8	2·8	0
120	55	4·1	0	0	0·50	0·10	1·0	2·8	0
121	4	0·4	0	0	0·08	0·03	1·5	1·5	0
122	23	1·2	0	0	0·09	0·06	1·7	1·8	0
123	14	0·5	0	0	0·01	0·02	0·1	0·1	206
124	25	12·0	2	0	0·03	0·09	0·5	1·4	0
125	52	15·0	7	0	0·08	0·30	1·7	4·8	0
126	0	0	0	0	0	0·20 (i)	10·0 (i)	10·0 (i)	0
127	140	4·0	0	0	0	0·10	45·0	45·7	0
128	0	0	0	0	0	0·90 (i)	6·0 (i)	6·0 (i)	0
129	10	0	0	0	0	0·05	0·7	0·7	0
130	0	0	0	0	0	0	0	0	0
131	6	0·8	0	0	0·01	0·02	0·2	0·2	0
132	42	0·8	2	0	0·08	0·02	0·6	0·9	2
133	88	1·8	24	0·27	0·14	0·10	1·8	2·1	0
134	71	1·8	56	0·80	0·70	0·70	0·3	1·2	0
135	50	1·3	0	0	0·06	0·01	0·6	0·8	0
136	67	1·4	82	1·20	0·70	0·10	0·7	1·8	0
137	116	0·1	96	0·08	0·05	0·14	0·2	1·0	1
138	18	0·3	46	0	0·03	0·02	0·5	0·2	6
139	75	0·6	73	0·30	0·04	0·10	0·3	1·1	2

(i) 90 to 100% is extracted into an infusion.

TABLE 2

Composition of foods per oz

No.	Food	Inedible waste	Energy value		Protein	Fat	Carbohydrate (as monosaccharide)
		%	kcal	kJ	g	g	g
	Milk						
1	Cream, double	0	128	534	0·5	13·6	0·7
2	Cream, single	0	54	225	0·8	5·1	1·2
3	Milk, liquid, whole	0	18	77	0·9	1·1	1·4
4	Milk, condensed, whole, sweetened	0	91	382	2·3	2·6	15·6
5	Milk, whole, evaporated	0	47	197	2·4	2·6	3·6
6	Milk, dried, whole	0	139	584	7·6	7·7	10·6
7	Milk, dried, half-cream	0	120	503	8·9	4·2	12·4
8	Milk, dried, skimmed	0	93	390	10·6	0·1	13·3
9	Yoghurt, natural	0	16	67	1·0	0·7	1·5
10	Yoghurt, fruit	0	22	92	1·0	0·5	3·7
	Cheese						
11	Cheese, Cheddar	0	117	490	7·2	9·8	0
12	Cheese, cottage	0	32	137	4·3	1·1	1·3
	Meat						
13	Bacon, average	13	135	566	3·1	13·6	0
14	Beef, average	17	89	373	4·2	8·0	0
15	Beef, corned	0	64	267	6·3	4·3	0
16	Beef, stewing steak, raw	0	60	252	4·8	4·5	0
17	Beef, stewing steak, cooked	0	69	288	8·2	4·0	0
18	Chicken, raw	31	41	171	5·9	1·9	0
19	Chicken, roast	—	52	219	8·4	2·1	0
20	Ham, cooked	0	119	500	4·6	11·2	0
21	Kidney, average	0	30	125	4·8	1·2	0
22	Lamb, average, raw	17	94	394	3·7	8·8	0
23	Lamb, roast	—	81	338	7·1	5·8	0
24	Liver, average, raw	0	39	165	4·7	2·3	0
25	Liver, fried	0	78	328	8·4	4·5	1·1
26	Luncheon meat	0	92	387	3·2	8·2	1·4
27	Pork, average	15	116	486	3·4	11·4	0
28	Pork, chop, grilled	40	150	627	5·3	14·3	0
29	Sausage, pork	0	105	439	2·9	8·8	3·8
30	Steak and Kidney pie, cooked	0	86	361	3·8	6·0	4·6
31	Tripe	0	17	71	3·3	0·3	0
	Fish						
32	Cod, haddock, white fish	40	19	82	4·5	0·1	0
33	Cod, fried in batter	0	56	236	5·6	2·9	2·1

TABLE 2—*contd.*

Composition per oz

No.	Calcium	Iron	Vitamin A (retinol equivalents)	Vitamin D	Thiamine	Riboflavine	Nicotinic acid Total	Nicotinic acid Equivalents	Vitamin C
	mg	mg	µg	µg	mg	mg	mg	mg	mg
1	18	0	119	0·08	0·01	0·02	0	0·1	0
2	28	0	44	0·03	0·01	0·04	0	0·2	0
3	34	0	12 (a) 10 (b)	0·01 (a) 0 (b)	0·01	0·04	0	0·3	1 (e)
4	82	0·1	32	0·04	0·03	0·11	0·1	0·6	1
5	82	0·1	32	0·04	0·02	0·11	0·1	0·6	0
6	230	0·2	70	0·08 (c) 2·50 (d)	0·09	0·31	0·2	2·0	3
7	266	0·2	41	0·05 (c) 2·50 (d)	0·10	0·38	0·3	2·3	3
8	362	0·3	1	0	0·09	0·49	0·3	2·8	3
9	40	0	11	0·01	0·01	0·05	0	0·3	0
10	40	0	6	0	0·01	0·05	0	0·3	0
11	230	0·2	119	0·10	0·01	0·14	0	1·5	0
12	23	0·1	8	0·01	0·01	0·08	0	0·9	0
13	3	0·3	0	0	0·11	0·04	0·4	1·1	0
14	3	1·1	0	0	0·02	0·06	1·4	2·2	0
15	4	2·8	0	0	0	0·06	1·0	2·2	0
16	3	1·1	0	0	0·02	0·06	1·4	2·3	0
17	2	1·4	0	0	0·01	0·06	1·4	3·0	0
18	3	0·4	0	0	0·01	0·05	1·7	2·7	0
19	4	0·7	0	0	0·01	0·04	1·4	2·8	0
20	4	0·7	0	0	0·14	0·06	1·0	2·0	0
21	4	3·8	85	0	0·09	0·57	2·0	3·2	3
22	3	0·6	0	0	0·04	0·07	1·4	2·2	0
23	1	1·2	0	0	0·03	0·07	1·3	2·8	0
24	2	3·9	1,701	0·21	0·09	0·85	3·7	4·9	9
25	3	5·9	1,701	0·21	0·09	0·99	4·3	6·4	6
26	5	0·3	0	0	0·11	0·06	1·0	1·7	0
27	3	0·3	0	0	0·28	0·06	1·4	2·2	0
28	2	0·7	0	0	0·23	0·06	1·4	2·6	0
29	4	0·7	0	0	0·05	0·02	0·5	1·1	0
30	10	1·4	36	0·16	0·03	0·13	1·2	1·7	0
31	20	0·2	3	0	0·05	0·03	1·0	1·6	0
32	7	0·3	0	0	0·02	0·03	0·8	1·7	0
33	23	0·1	0	0	0·01	0·03	0·8	1·9	0

(a) Summer value. (b) Winter value. (c) Natural value. (d) With fortification.
(e) Less than 1 mg.

TABLE 2—*contd.*

Composition per oz

No.	Food	Inedible waste	Energy value		Protein	Fat	Carbohydrate (as monosaccharide)
		%	kcal	kJ	g	g	g
	Fish contd.:						
34	Fish fingers . .	0	54	228	3·8	1·9	5·9
35	Herring . .	37	54	226	4·5	4·0	0
36	Kipper . . .	40	62	261	5·4	4·5	0
37	Salmon, canned .	2	38	158	5·6	1·7	0
38	Sardines, canned in oil . . .	0	81	339	5·8	6·4	0
	Eggs						
39	Eggs, fresh . .	12	45	188	3·4	3·5	0
	Fats						
40	Butter . . .	0	211	884	0·1	23·4	0
41	Lard, cooking fat, dripping . .	0	253	1,064	0	28·2	0
42	Margarine . .	0	218	913	0·1	24·2	0
43	Oils, cooking and salad . . .	0	255	1,070	0	28·3	0
	Preserves etc.						
44	Chocolate, milk .	0	164	687	2·5	10·7	15·5
45	Honey . . .	0	82	344	0·1	0	21·7
46	Jam . . .	0	74	310	0·1	0	19·6
47	Ice cream, vanilla .	0	55	230	1·2	3·2	5·6
48	Marmalade . .	0	74	310	0	0	19·7
49	Sugar, white . .	0	112	469	0	0	29·8
50	Syrup . . .	0	84	352	0·1	0	22·4
	Vegetables						
51	Beans, canned in tomato sauce .	0	26	109	1·7	0·1	4·9
52	Beans, broad . .	75	19	80	2·0	0·1	2·7
53	Beans, haricot .	0	73	305	6·1	0	12·9
54	Beans, runner .	14	4	18	0·3	0	0·8
55	Beetroot, boiled .	20	12	52	0·5	0	2·8
56	Brussels sprouts, raw	25	9	38	1·0	0	1·3
57	Brussels sprouts, boiled . . .	0	5	19	0·7	0	0·5
58	Cabbage, raw .	30	8	33	0·4	0	1·6
59	Cabbage, boiled .	0	2	9	0·2	0	0·4
60	Carrots, old . .	4	7	27	0·2	0	1·5
61	Cauliflower . .	30	7	29	1·0	0	0·8
62	Celery . . .	27	2	9	0·3	0	0·4
63	Lentils, dry . .	0	84	351	6·8	0	15·1
64	Lettuce . .	20	3	13	0·3	0	0·5
65	Mushrooms . .	25	2	8	0·5	0	0
66	Onions . . .	3	7	27	0·3	0	1·5
67	Parsnips . .	26	14	58	0·5	0	3·2
68	Peas, fresh, raw or quick frozen .	63 / 0	18	75	1·6	0	3·0

TABLE 2—*contd.*

Composition per oz

No.	Calcium	Iron	Vitamin A (retinol equivalents)	Vitamin D	Thiamine	Riboflavine	Nicotinic acid Total	Nicotinic acid Equivalents	Vitamin C
	mg	mg	μg	μg	mg	mg	mg	mg	mg
34	14	0·4	0	0	0·03	0·05	0·5	1·1	0
35	28	0·4	13	6·38	0·01	0·09	1·0	1·8	0
36	34	0·6	13	6·38	0	0·09	1·0	2·0	0
37	19	0·4	26	3·54	0·01	0·03	2·0	3·0	0
38	116	1·1	9	2·12	0	0·06	1·4	2·5	0
39	16	0·7	85	0·43	0·03	0·10	0	0·9	0
40	4	0	282	0·36	0	0	0	0	0
41	0	0	0	0	0	0	0	0	0
42	1	0·1	255 (e)	2·27	0	0	0	0	0
43	0	0	0	0	0	0	0	0	0
44	70	0·5	2	0	0·01	0·10	0·3	0·7	0
45	1	0·1	0	0	0	0·01	0·1	0·1	0
46	5	0·3	1	0	0	0	0	0	3
47	39	0·1	0	0	0·01	0·06	0	0·3	0
48	10	0·2	2	0	0	0	0	0	3
49	0	0	0	0	0	0	0	0	0
50	7	0·4	0	0	0	0	0	0	0
51	18	0·6	14	0	0·02	0·01	0·1	0·4	1
52	9	0·3	6	0	0·08	0·01	1·1	1·4	9
53	51	1·9	0	0	0·13	0·04	0·7	1·7	0
54	9	0·2	14	0	0·01	0·03	0·3	0·4	6
55	9	0·2	0	0	0	0·01	0	0·1	1
56	8	0·2	19	0	0·03	0·05	0·2	0·4	28
57	8	0·2	19	0	0·02	0·03	0·1	0·3	10
58	18	0·3	14	0	0·02	0·01	0·1	0·1	17
59	16	0·1	14	0	0·01	0·01	0·1	0·1	6
60	14	0·2	567	0	0·02	0·01	0·2	0·2	2
61	5	0·2	1	0	0·03	0·03	0·2	0·4	20
62	15	0·2	0	0	0·01	0·01	0·1	0·1	2
63	11	2·2	2	0	0·14	0·07	0·7	1·8	0
64	7	0·2	47	0	0·02	0·02	0·1	0·1	4
65	1	0·3	0	0	0·03	0·11	1·1	1·2	1
66	9	0·1	0	0	0·01	0·01	0·1	0·1	3
67	16	0·2	0	0	0·03	0·03	0·3	0·4	4
68	4	0·5	14	0	0·09	0·04	0·7	1·0	7

(e) some margarines contain carotene.

TABLE 2—*contd.*

Composition per oz

No.	Food	Inedible waste	Energy value		Protein	Fat	Carbo-hydrate (as mono-saccharide)
		%	kcal	kJ	g	g	g
	Vegetables contd.:						
69	Peas, fresh boiled or quick frozen boiled.		14	58	1·4	0	2·2
70	Peas, canned, processed . .	0	27	114	2·0	0	5·1
71	Peppers, green .	18	6	25	0·3	0·1	1·1
72	Potatoes, raw .	27 (f) 14 (g)	22	91	0·6	0	5·1
73	Potatoes, boiled .	0	23	94	0·4	0	5·6
74	Potato chips, fried .	0	67	281	1·1	2·6	10·6
75	Potatoes, roast .	0	35	146	0·8	0·3	7·7
76	Spinach . .	25	6	25	0·8	0	0·8
77	Sweet corn, canned	0	27	113	0·7	0·2	5·8
78	Tomatoes, fresh .	0	4	17	0·3	0	0·8
79	Turnips . .	16	5	20	0·2	0	1·1
80	Watercress . .	23	4	17	0·8	0	0·2
	Fruit						
81	Apple . . .	25	13	55	0·1	0	3·4
82	Apricots, canned .	0	30	126	0·1	0	7·9
83	Apricots, dried .	0	52	217	1·4	0	12·3
84	Bananas . .	40	22	90	0·3	0	5·5
85	Black currants .	2	8	33	0·3	0	1·9
86	Cherries . .	15	13	55	0·2	0	3·4
87	Dates . . .	14	70	295	0·6	0	18·1
88	Figs, dried . .	0	60	253	1·0	0	15·0
89	Gooseberries. .	0	8	32	0·3	0	1·8
90	Grapefruit . .	50	6	26	0·2	0	1·5
91	Lemons . .	64	2	8	0·1	0	0·5
92	Melon . . .	41	7	27	0·2	0	1·5
93	Oranges . .	25	10	42	0·2	0	2·4
94	Orange juice, canned, unconcen-trated . . .	0	13	54	0·2	0	3·3
95	Peaches, fresh .	13	11	44	0·2	0	2·6
96	Peaches, canned .	0	25	105	0·1	0	6·5
97	Pears, fresh . .	25	12	49	0·1	0	3·0
98	Pineapple, canned .	0	22	90	0·1	0	5·7
99	Plums . . .	8	9	38	0·2	0	2·2
100	Prunes. . . .	17	46	192	0·7	0	11·4
101	Raspberries . .	0	7	30	0·3	0	1·6
102	Rhubarb . .	33	2	7	0·2	0	0·3
103	Strawberries . .	3	7	31	0·2	0	1·8
104	Sultanas . .	0	71	296	0·5	0	18·3
	Nuts						
105	Almonds . .	63	164	688	5·8	15·2	1·2
106	Coconut, desiccated	0	172	722	1·9	17·6	1·8
107	Peanuts, roasted .	0	166	697	8·0	13·9	2·4

(f) old potatoes. (g) new potatoes.

TABLE 2—*contd.*

Composition per oz

No.	Calcium	Iron	Vitamin A (retinol equivalents)	Vitamin D	Thiamine	Riboflavine	Nicotinic acid		Vitamin C
							Total	Equivalents	
	mg	mg	µg	µg	mg	mg	mg	mg	mg
69	4	0·3	14	0	0·07	0·03	0·4	0·7	4
70	8	0·3	19	0	0·02	0·01	0·1	0·4	1
71	3	0·2	12	0	0·02	0·02	0·1	0·2	36
72	2	0·2	0	0	0·03	0·01	0·3	0·5	2–9 (h)
73	1	0·1	0	0	0·02	0·01	0·2	0·3	1–4 (h)
74	4	0·4	0	0	0·03	0·01	0·3	0·6	2–6 (h)
75	3	0·3	0	0	0·03	0·02	0·3	0·6	2–7 (h)
76	20	0·9	284	0	0·03	0·06	0·2	0·4	17
77	1	0·1	10	0	0·01	0·01	0·3	0·1	1
78	4	0·1	33	0	0·02	0·01	0·2	0·2	6
79	17	0·1	0	0	0·01	0·01	0·2	0·2	7
80	63	0·5	142	0	0·03	0·05	0·2	0·6	17
81	1	0·1	1	0	0·01	0·01	0	0	1
82	3	0·2	47	0	0·01	0	0·1	0·1	1
83	26	1·2	170	0	0	0·06	0·9	1·0	0
84	2	0·1	9	0	0·01	0·02	0·2	0·2	3
85	17	0·4	9	0	0·01	0·02	0·1	0·1	57
86	5	0·1	6	0	0·01	0·02	0·1	0·1	1
87	19	0·5	3	0	0·02	0·01	0·6	0·7	0
88	81	1·2	2	0	0·03	0·04	0·5	0·6	0
89	6	0·1	9	0	0·01	0·01	0·1	0·1	11
90	5	0·1	0	0	0·01	0·01	0·1	0·1	11
91	2	0	0	0	0·01	0	0	0	14
92	5	0·1	45	0	0·01	0·01	0·1	0·1	7
93	12	0·1	2	0	0·03	0·01	0·1	0·1	14
94	3	0·1	2	0	0·02	0·01	0·1	0·1	11
95	1	0·1	24	0	0·01	0·01	0·3	0·3	2
96	1	0·5	12	0	0	0·01	0·2	0·2	1
97	2	0·1	1	0	0·01	0·01	0·1	0·1	1
98	4	0·5	2	0	0·01	0·01	0·1	0·1	2
99	3	0·1	10	0	0·01	0·01	0·1	0·2	1
100	11	0·8	45	0	0·03	0·06	0·4	0·5	0
101	12	0·3	4	0	0·01	0·01	0·1	0·1	7
102	29	0·1	3	0	0	0·02	0·1	0·1	3
103	6	0·2	1	0	0·01	0·01	0·1	0·1	17
104	15	0·5	0	0	0·03	0·09	0·1	0·2	0
105	70	1·2	0	0	0·09	0·07	0·6	1·4	0
106	6	1·0	0	0	0·02	0·01	0·2	0·5	0
107	17	0·6	0	0	0·07	0·03	4·5	5·9	0

(h) vitamin C falls during storage.

TABLE 2—*contd.*

Composition per oz

No.	Food	Inedible waste	Energy value		Protein	Fat	Carbo-hydrate (as mono-saccharide)
		%	kcal	kJ	g	g	g
	Cereals						
108	Barley, pearl, dry .	0	102	428	2·2	0·5	23·7
109	Biscuits, chocolate .	0	142	595	2·0	7·1	18·5
110	Biscuits, plain, semi-sweet . . .	0	122	511	2·1	3·7	21·3
111	Biscuits, rich, sweet	0	141	591	1·6	6·3	20·6
112	Bread, brown .	0	66	277	2·6	0·5	13·7
113	Bread, starch reduced . .	0	66	278	3·0	0·4	13·5
114	Bread, white. .	0	72	302	2·4	0·5	15·5
115	Bread, wholemeal .	0	68	285	2·7	0·9	13·2
116	Cornflakes . .	0	103	432	2·1	0·1	24·9
117	Custard powder, instant pudding, cornflour . .	0	100	420	0·1	0·2	26·1
118	Crispbread, Ryvita	0	90	378	2·8	0·6	19·6
119	Flour, white . .	0	99	414	2·8	0·3	22·7
120	Oatmeal . .	0	113	475	3·4	2·5	20·6
121	Rice . . .	0	102	427	1·8	0·3	24·6
122	Spaghetti . .	0	103	432	2·8	0·3	23·8
	Beverages						
123	Black currant juice	0	65	272	0·1	0	17·3
124	Chocolate, drinking	0	116	487	1·6	1·9	25·0
125	Cocoa powder .	0	126	530	5·3	6·4	12·8
126	Coffee, ground .	0	0	0	0	0	0
127	Coffee, instant .	0	44	184	1·1	0·2	10·1
128	Tea, dry . .	0	0	0	0	0	0
	Alcoholic Beverages						
129	Beer, mild, draught	0	7	29	0·1	0	0·5
130	Spirits, 70% proof .	0	63	264	0	0	0
131	Wine, red . .	0	19	80	0	0	0·1
	Puddings and Cakes etc.						
132	Apple pie . .	0	83	349	0·9	4·1	11·5
133	Buns, currant .	0	93	390	2·2	2·4	16·6
134	Fruit cake, rich .	0	104	436	1·3	4·5	15·6
135	Jam tarts . .	0	111	465	0·9	3·9	19·2
136	Plain cake, Madeira	0	122	511	1·7	6·8	14·1
137	Rice pudding .	0	41	169	1·0	2·2	4·5
138	Soup, tomato, canned. . .	0	19	80	0·3	0·9	2·7
139	Trifle . . .	0	46	193	0·9	1·6	7·5

TABLE 2—*contd.*

Composition per oz

No.	Calcium	Iron	Vitamin A (retinol equivalents)	Vitamin D	Thiamine	Riboflavine	Nicotinic acid		Vitamin C
							Total	Equivalents	
	mg	mg	μg	μg	mg	mg	mg	mg	mg
108	3	0·2	0	0	0·03	0·02	0·7	0·6	0
109	37	0·4	0	0	0·03	0·01	0·3	0·6	0
110	36	0·5	0	0	0·05	0·02	0·4	0·6	0
111	26	0·4	0	0	0·03	0·01	0·3	0·4	0
112	26	0·7	0	0	0·08	0·02	0·9	0·7	0
113	28	0·4	0	0	0·05	0·01	0·4	0·8	0
114	28	0·5	0	0	0·05	0	0·4	0·7	0
115	8	0·9	0	0	0·07	0·03	0·7	0·5	0
116	1	0·3	0	0	0·17	0·30	2·0	1·8	0
117	4	0·4	0	0	0	0	0	0	0
118	24	0·9	0	0	0·10	0·07	0·4	0·4	0
119	41	0·5	0	0	0·08	0·01	0·5	0·8	0
120	16	1·2	0	0	0·14	0·03	0·3	0·8	0
121	1	0·1	0	0	0·02	0·01	0·4	0·4	0
122	6	0·3	0	0	0·03	0·02	0·5	0·5	0
123	4	0·1	0	0	0	0·01	0	0	58
124	7	3·4	1	0	0·01	0·03	0·1	0·4	0
125	15	4·3	2	0	0·02	0·01	0·5	1·4	0
126	0	0	0	0	0	0·06 (i)	2·8 (i)	2·8 (i)	0
127	40	1·1	0	0	0	0·03	12·8	12·9	0
128	0	0	0	0	0	0·30 (i)	1·7 (i)	1·7 (i)	0
129	3	0	0	0	0	0·01	0·2	0·2	0
130	0	0	0	0	0	0	0	0	0
131	2	0·2	0	0	0	0	0	0	0
132	12	0·2	4	0	0·02	0·01	0·2	0·3	1
133	25	0·5	7	0·80	0·04	0·03	0·5	0·6	0
134	20	0·5	16	0·23	0·02	0·02	0·1	0·3	0
135	14	0·4	0	0	0·02	0	0·2	0·2	0
136	19	0·4	23	0·34	0·02	0·03	0·2	0·5	0
137	33	0	27	0·02	0·01	0·04	0·1	0·3	0
138	5	0·1	13	0	0·01	0·01	0·1	0·1	2
139	21	0·2	21	0·08	0·01	0·03	0·1	0·3	1

(i) 90–100% extracted into an infusion.

Table 3

Composition of foods per 100 kcal

No.	Food	Protein	Fat	Carbohydrate (as monosaccharide)	Calcium	Iron
		g	g	g	mg	mg
	Milk					
1	Cream, double	0·4	10·7	0·6	14	0
2	Cream, single	1·5	9·5	2·2	53	0·1
3	Milk, liquid, whole	5·1	5·8	7·4	185	0·2
4	Milk, condensed, whole, sweetened	2·5	2·9	17·1	90	0·1
5	Milk, whole, evaporated	5·1	5·5	7·7	175	0·1
6	Milk, dried, whole	5·4	5·5	7·6	165	0·1
7	Milk, dried, half-cream	7·4	4·0	10·3	221	0·2
8	Milk, dried, skimmed	11·3	0·2	14·3	388	0·3
9	Yoghurt, natural	6·3	4·6	9·2	246	0·2
10	Yoghurt, fruit	4·6	2·3	16·4	177	0·1
	Cheese					
11	Cheese, Cheddar	6·2	8·4	0	197	0·1
12	Cheese, cottage	13·3	3·5	3·8	70	0·3
	Meat					
13	Bacon, average	2·3	10·1	0	2	0·2
14	Beef, average	4·7	9·0	0	3	1·3
15	Beef, corned	10·0	6·7	0	6	4·4
16	Beef, stewing steak, raw	8·0	7·5	0	5	1·9
17	Beef, stewing steak, cooked	12·0	5·8	0	3	2·1
18	Chicken, raw	14·4	4·7	0	8	1·0
19	Chicken, roast	16·1	4·0	0	8	1·4
20	Ham, cooked	3·9	9·3	0	3	0·6
21	Kidney, average	16·1	4·0	0	13	12·8
22	Lamb, average, raw	3·9	9·4	0	3	0·6
23	Lamb, roast	8·8	7·2	0	1	1·5
24	Liver, average, raw	11·9	5·8	0	6	10·0
25	Liver, fried	10·7	5·8	1·4	3	7·5
26	Luncheon meat	3·5	8·9	1·5	6	0·3
27	Pork, average	2·9	9·8	0	2	0·2
28	Pork chop, grilled	3·5	9·5	0	2	0·5
29	Sausage, pork	2·8	8·4	3·6	4	0·7
30	Steak and kidney pie, cooked	4·4	6·9	5·3	12	1·7
31	Tripe	19·3	1·7	0	117	1·2
	Fish					
32	Cod, haddock, white fish	23·2	0·7	0	36	1·4
33	Cod, fried in batter	9·8	5·2	3·8	40	0·3

TABLE 3—*contd.*

Composition per 100 kcal

No.	Vitamin A (retinol equivalents)	Vitamin D	Thiamine	Riboflavine	Nicotinic acid equivalents	Vitamin C
	μg	μg	mg	mg	mg	mg
1	94	0·06	0	0·02	0·1	0
2	82	0·05	0·02	0·07	0·4	0
3	68 (a) 57 (b)	0·07 (a) 0·02 (b)	0·06	0·23	1·4	2
4	35	0·04	0·03	0·12	0·6	1
5	67	0·08	0·04	0·22	1·2	1
6	50	0·06 (c) 1·79 (d)	0·06	0·20	1·4	2
7	34	0·04 (c) 2·08 (d)	0·08	0·32	1·9	2
8	1	0	0·09	0·53	2·9	3
9	68	0·04	0·09	0·33	1·6	0
10	28	0·02	0·06	0·24	1·1	0
11	102	0·08	0·01	0·12	1·3	0
12	23	0·02	0·03	0·23	2·8	0
13	0	0	0·08	0·03	0·8	0
14	0	0	0·02	0·06	2·5	0
15	0	0	0	0·09	3·4	0
16	0	0	0·03	0·09	3·9	0
17	0	0	0·02	0·09	4·3	0
18	0	0	0·03	0·12	6·6	0
19	0	0	0·02	0·08	5·4	0
20	0	0	0·11	0·05	1·7	0
21	286	0	0·30	1·90	10·6	11
22	0	0	0·05	0·08	2·3	0
23	0	0	0·04	0·09	3·5	0
24	4,317	0·54	0·22	2·20	12·3	22
25	2,174	0·27	0·11	1·27	8·1	7
26	0	0	0·12	0·06	1·8	0
27	0	0	0·20	0·05	1·9	0
28	0	0	0·15	0·04	1·7	0
29	0	0	0·05	0·02	1·6	0
30	41	0·18	0·04	0·15	2·0	0
31	17	0	0·30	0·17	9·5	0
32	0	0	0·09	0·14	8·7	0
33	0	0	0·02	0·05	3·3	0

(a) Summer value. (b) Winter value. (c) Natural value. (d) With fortification.

TABLE 3—*contd.*

Composition per 100 *kcal*

No.	Food	Protein	Fat	Carbohydrate (as monosaccharide)	Calcium	Iron
		g	g	g	mg	mg
	Fish contd.:					
34	Fish fingers	7·0	3·5	10·8	26	0·7
35	Herring	8·4	7·4	0	53	0·8
36	Kipper	8·6	7·3	0	54	0·9
37	Salmon, canned	14·8	4·5	0	50	1·0
38	Sardines, canned in oil	7·2	7·9	0	144	1·4
	Eggs					
39	Eggs, fresh	7·5	7·8	0	35	1·6
	Fats					
40	Butter	0·1	11·1	0	2	0
41	Lard, cooking fat, dripping	0	11·1	0	0	0
42	Margarine	0	11·1	0	1	0
43	Oils, cooking and salad	0	11·1	0	0	0
	Preserves etc.					
44	Chocolate, milk	1·5	6·5	9·4	43	0·3
45	Honey	0·1	0	26·5	2	0·1
46	Jam	0·2	0	26·4	7	0·5
47	Ice cream, vanilla	2·1	5·9	10·3	71	0·2
48	Marmalade	0	0	26·6	13	0·2
49	Sugar, white	0	0	26·6	0	0
50	Syrup	0·1	0	26·6	9	0·5
	Vegetables					
51	Beans, canned in tomato sauce	6·5	0·4	18·8	67	2·3
52	Beans, broad	10·4	0·7	13·8	43	1·6
53	Beans, haricot	8·4	0	17·8	70	2·6
54	Beans, runner	7·3	0	19·3	220	4·7
55	Beetroot, boiled	4·1	0	22·5	68	1·6
56	Brussels sprouts, raw	11·3	0	14·4	91	2·2
57	Brussels sprouts, boiled	15·0	0	10·6	169	3·8
58	Cabbage, raw	5·4	0	20·7	232	3·6
59	Cabbage, boiled	10·0	0	16·3	725	6·3
60	Carrots, old	3·0	0	23·5	209	2·6
61	Cauliflower	14·2	0	11·7	75	2·5
62	Celery	11·3	0	16·3	650	7·5
63	Lentils, dry	8·1	0	18·0	13	2·6
64	Lettuce	10·0	0	16·4	236	6·4
65	Mushrooms	25·7	0	0	43	14·3
66	Onions	3·9	0	22·6	135	1·3
67	Parsnips	3·5	0	23·1	112	1·2
68	Peas, fresh raw or quick frozen	9·2	0	16·8	24	3·0
69	Peas, fresh, boiled or quick frozen boiled	10·2	0	15·7	27	2·4

TABLE 3—*contd.*

Composition per 100 *kcal*

No.	Vitamin A (retinol equivalents)	Vitamin D	Thiamine	Riboflavine	Nicotinic acid equivalents	Vitamin C
	µg	µg	mg	mg	mg	mg
34	0	0	0·06	0·08	2·0	0
35	24	11·71	0·02	0·16	3·4	0
36	20	10·11	0	0·14	3·1	0
37	68	9·40	0·02	0·08	8·0	0
38	11	2·63	0	0·07	3·0	0
39	190	0·95	0·06	0·22	1·9	0
40	134	0·17	0	0	0	0
41	0	0	0	0	0	0
42	117 (e)	1·04	0	0	0	0
43	0	0	0	0	0	0
44	1	0	0·01	0·06	0·4	0
45	0	0	0	0·02	0·1	0
46	1	0	0	0	0	4
47	1	0	0·03	0·10	0·6	1
48	3	0	0	0	0	4
49	0	0	0	0	0	0
50	0	0	0	0	0	0
51	54	0	0·07	0·04	1·6	3
52	32	0	0·41	0·07	7·2	43
53	0	0	0·18	0·05	2·4	0
54	333	0	0·33	0·67	8·0	133
55	0	0	0·05	0·09	0·9	11
56	209	0	0·31	0·50	4·4	313
57	419	0	0·38	0·63	5·6	219
58	179	0	0·21	0·18	1·8	214
59	625	0	0·38	0·38	3·8	250
60	8,698	0	0·26	0·22	3·0	26
61	21	0	0·42	0·42	5·8	292
62	0	0	0·38	0·38	6·3	88
63	2	0	0·17	0·08	2·2	0
64	1,518	0	0·64	0·73	3·6	136
65	0	0	1·43	5·71	64·3	43
66	0	0	0·13	0·22	1·7	43
67	0	0	0·20	0·18	2·7	31
68	79	0	0·51	0·24	5·6	40
69	102	0	0·51	0·22	4·7	31

(e) some margarines contain carotene.

TABLE 3—*contd.*

Composition per 100 kcal

No.	Food	Protein	Fat	Carbo-hydrate (as mono-saccharide)	Calcium	Iron
		g	g	g	mg	mg
	Vegetables contd.:					
70	Peas, canned, processed .	7·5	0	18·8	30	1·1
71	Peppers, green . .	5·7	1·0	17·6	43	3·3
72	Potatoes, raw . . .	2·8	0	23·7	11	0·9
73	Potatoes, boiled . .	1·8	0	24·9	5	0·6
74	Potato chips, fried . .	1·6	3·8	15·8	6	0·6
75	Potatoes, roast . .	2·3	0·8	2·2	8	0·8
76	Spinach. . . .	12·9	0	13·3	333	15·2
77	Sweet corn, canned. .	2·7	0·8	21·6	5	0·5
78	Tomatoes, fresh . .	6·4	0	20·0	93	2·9
79	Turnips. . . .	4·7	0	22·4	347	2·4
80	Watercress . . .	20·7	0	5·0	1,586	11·4
	Fruit					
81	Apple	0·7	0	26·1	9	0·7
82	Apricots, canned . .	0·5	0	26·1	11	0·7
83	Apricots, dried . .	2·6	0	23·8	51	2·3
84	Bananas. . . .	1·4	0	25·3	9	0·5
85	Black currants . .	3·2	0	23·6	214	4·6
86	Cherries. . . .	1·3	0	25·7	39	0·9
87	Dates	0·8	0	25·8	27	0·6
88	Figs, dried . . .	1·7	0	24·8	133	2·0
89	Gooseberries . . .	3·3	0	23·3	81	1·7
90	Grapefruit . . .	2·7	0	24·1	77	1·4
91	Lemons	4·3	0	22·9	114	2·0
92	Melon	3·5	0	22·6	70	2·2
93	Oranges. . . .	2·3	0	24·3	117	0·9
94	Orange juice, canned, un-concentrated . . .	1·7	0	24·9	21	0·9
95	Peaches, fresh. . .	1·6	0	24·6	14	1·1
96	Peaches, canned . .	0·5	0	26·0	4	2·2
97	Pears, fresh . . .	0·7	0	25·9	20	0·5
98	Pineapple, canned . .	0·4	0	26·3	17	2·2
99	Plums	1·9	0	24·7	38	0·9
100	Prunes	1·5	0	25·0	24	1·8
101	Raspberries . . .	3·6	0	22·4	164	4·8
102	Rhubarb . . .	10·0	0	16·7	1,717	6·7
103	Strawberries . . .	2·3	0	23·8	85	2·7
104	Sultanas . . .	0·7	0	26·0	21	0·7
	Nuts					
105	Almonds	3·5	9·2	0·7	43	0·7
106	Coconut, desiccated. .	1·1	10·2	1·1	4	0·6
107	Peanuts, roasted . .	4·8	8·4	1·5	10	0·3
	Cereals					
108	Barley, pearl, dry . .	2·1	0·5	23·2	3	0·2
109	Biscuits, chocolate . .	1·4	5·0	13·1	26	0·3

TABLE 3—*contd.*

Composition per 100 *kcal*

No.	Vitamin A (retinol equivalents)	Vitamin D	Thiamine	Riboflavine	Nicotinic acid equivalents	Vitamin C
	μg	μg	mg	mg	mg	mg
70	70	0	0·06	0·05	1·6	2
71	200	0	0·38	0·38	3·3	610
72	0	0	0·14	0·05	2·4	10–40 (f)
73	0	0	0·10	0·04	1·5	5–19 (f)
74	0	0	0·04	0·02	0·9	2–8 (f)
75	0	0	0·08	0·03	1·6	5–19 (f)
76	4,762	0	0·57	0·95	6·2	286
77	37	0	0·03	0·05	0·3	4
78	836	0	0·43	0·29	5·0	143
79	0	0	0·24	0·29	4·7	147
80	3,571	0	0·71	1·14	14·3	429
81	11	0	0·09	0·04	0·2	11
82	156	0	0·02	0·01	0·3	5
83	330	0	0	0·10	1·9	0
84	43	0	0·05	0·09	1·1	13
85	118	0	0·11	0·21	1·1	714
86	43	0	0·11	0·13	0·9	11
87	4	0	0·03	0·02	0·9	0
88	4	0	0·05	0·06	1·0	0
89	111	0	0·15	0·11	1·5	148
90	0	0	0·23	0·09	1·4	182
91	0	0	0·29	0	1·4	714
92	696	0	0·22	0·13	2·2	109
93	23	0	0·29	0·09	0·9	143
94	17	0	0·15	0·04	0·4	85
95	224	0	0·05	0·14	3·0	22
96	48	0	0·01	0·02	0·7	5
97	5	0	0·07	0·07	0·7	7
98	9	0	0·07	0·03	0·4	11
99	116	0	0·16	0·09	1·9	9
100	99	0	0·06	0·12	1·1	0
101	52	0	0·08	0·12	2·0	100
102	167	0	0	1·17	5·0	167
103	19	0	0·08	0·12	1·9	231
104	0	0	0·04	0·12	0·2	0
105	0	0	0·06	0·04	0·8	0
106	0	0	0·01	0·01	0·3	0
107	0	0	0·04	0·02	3·5	0
108	0	0	0·03	0·02	0·6	0
109	0	0	0·02	0·01	0·4	0

(f) vitamin C falls during storage.

TABLE 3—*contd.*

Composition per 100 kcal

No.	Food	Protein	Fat	Carbo-hydrate (as mono-saccharide)	Calcium	Iron
		g	g	g	mg	mg
	Cereals contd.:					
110	Biscuits, plain, semi-sweet	1·7	3·1	17·5	29	0·4
111	Biscuits, rich, sweet . .	1·1	4·5	14·7	19	0·3
112	Bread, brown . . .	3·9	0·8	21·0	39	1·1
113	Bread, starch reduced .	4·3	0·6	20·5	43	0·6
114	Bread, white . . .	3·3	0·7	21·6	40	0·7
115	Bread, wholemeal . .	4·0	1·3	19·4	12	1·2
116	Cornflakes . . .	2·1	0·1	24·1	1	0·3
117	Custard powder, instant pudding, cornflour . .	0·1	0·2	26·1	4	0·4
118	Crispbread, Ryvita . .	3·1	0·7	22·0	27	1·0
119	Flour, white . . .	2·9	0·3	23·0	42	0·5
120	Oatmeal . . .	3·0	2·2	18·2	14	1·0
121	Rice	1·7	0·3	24·2	1	0·1
122	Spaghetti . . .	2·7	0·3	23·1	6	0·3
	Beverages					
123	Black currant juice . .	0·1	0	26·6	6	0·2
124	Chocolate, drinking. .	1·4	1·7	21·0	6	2·9
125	Cocoa powder . .	4·2	5·0	10·1	12	3·4
126	Coffee, ground . .	0	0	0	0	0
127	Coffee, instant . .	2·6	0·4	22·8	90	2·6
128	Tea, dry . . .	0	0	0	0	0
	Alcoholic Beverages					
129	Beer, mild, draught .	0·8	0	6·4	40	0
130	Spirits, 70% proof . .	0	0	0	0	0
131	Wine, red . . .	0·3	0	0·4	9	1·2
	Puddings and Cakes etc.					
132	Apple pie . . .	1·1	4·9	13·7	14	0·3
133	Buns, currant . . .	2·4	2·6	17·9	27	0·5
134	Fruit cake, rich . .	1·2	4·3	15·0	19	0·5
135	Jam tarts . . .	0·8	3·5	17·3	13	0·3
136	Plain cake, Madeira .	1·7	6·0	11·6	16	0·3
137	Rice pudding . . .	2·5	5·4	11·1	82	0·1
138	Soup, tomato, canned .	1·4	4·6	14·0	27	0·4
139	Trifle	1·9	3·5	16·4	46	0·4

TABLE 3—*contd.*

Composition per 100 *kcal*

No.	Vitamin A (retinol equivalents)	Vitamin D	Thiamine	Riboflavine	Nicotinic acid equivalents	Vitamin C
	µg	µg	mg	mg	mg	mg
110	0	0	0·04	0·01	0·5	0
111	0	0	0·02	0·01	0·3	0
112	0	0	0·12	0·03	1·1	0
113	0	0	0·08	0·01	1·2	0
114	0	0	0·07	0·01	0·9	0
115	0	0	0·10	0·04	0·8	0
116	0	0	0·16	0·29	1·8	0
117	0	0	0	0	0	0
118	0	0	0·10	0·08	0·4	0
119	0	0	0·08	0·01	0·8	0
120	0	0	0·13	0·03	0·7	0
121	0	0	0·02	0·01	0·4	0
122	0	0	0·02	0·02	0·5	0
123	0	0	0	0·01	0	90
124	1	0	0·01	0·02	0·4	0
125	2	0	0·02	0·01	1·1	0
126	0	0	0	0	0	0
127	0	0	0	0·06	29·2	0
128	0	0	0	0	0	0
129	0	0	0	0·20	2·8	0
130	0	0	0	0	0	0
131	0	0	0·01	0·03	0·3	0
132	1	0	0·03	0·01	0·3	1
133	7	0·08	0·04	0·03	0·6	0
134	15	0·20	0·20	0·20	0·3	0
135	0	0	0·02	0	0·2	0
136	19	0·30	0·16	0·02	0·4	0
137	67	0·06	0·04	0·10	0·7	1
138	68	0	0·04	0·03	0·3	8
139	45	0·20	0·02	0·06	0·7	1

Appendix B

SCHEME FOR LECTURES

PART I

LECTURE 1	Introduction to Nutrition Carbohydrates
LECTURE 2	Fats Proteins
LECTURE 3	Food Consumption and Physical Work

PART II

LECTURE 4	Calcium and Phosphorus Iron Other Inorganic Elements
LECTURE 5	Vitamin A Vitamins D, E and K
LECTURE 6	The Vitamin B Group of Nutrients Vitamin C

PART III

LECTURE 7	Digestion of Foods and Absorption of Nutrients
LECTURE 8	Recommended Nutrient Intakes
LECTURE 9	Composition of Food

PART IV

LECTURE 10	Cooking
LECTURE 11	Meals
LECTURE 12	Planning Balanced Meals

Appendix C

SUGGESTED DEMONSTRATIONS

CARBOHYDRATES, FATS, PROTEINS

Examine and taste glucose, lactose, maltose and sucrose.
Examine under the microscope (if the students have had previous experience with this instrument) starch from potato, flour, cornflour, rice, etc., cooked and raw.
Demonstrate grams and ounces and calculate weights in grams and ounces.
Demonstrate by dissection the amount of fat in two pieces of meat.
Demonstrate saponification of animal fat and resistance to saponification of mineral wax.
Compare the properties of egg albumen, gelatin, gluten, casein and dried meat.

INORGANIC ELEMENTS AND VITAMINS

Weigh out amounts of cheese, milk, watercress, cabbage, potato and flour each containing 100 mg of calcium.
Weigh out 250 mg of chalk which also contains 100 mg of calcium.
Weigh out amounts of meat, bread and potato each containing 1 mg of iron.
Compare the amounts of vitamin A in the following meals by weighing the ingredients and calculating the vitamin A content in terms of retinol equivalents e.g.,
(1) Meat, potato, cabbage, steamed pudding;
(2) Bread, butter, cheese, milk, tomato.
Do a similar exercise for nicotinic acid, in terms of nicotinic acid equivalents.
Compare the amounts of thiamine, riboflavine, and nicotinic acid equivalents obtained from 4 oz of bread, oatmeal, peanuts, dried peas and milk. Weigh out sufficient potato, cabbage, lettuce, orange and apple to provide 20 mg of vitamin C.

DIGESTION OF FOODS AND ABSORPTION OF NUTRIENTS AND RECOMMENDED NUTRIENT INTAKES

Compare the result of a piece of meat shaken up in pepsin solution, with meat shaken up in water; similarly compare bread shaken up in saliva and fat shaken up with bile salts with the corresponding treatment using water alone.
Calculate the complete nutritional value of two diets provided, by weighing their ingredients and make suggestions for improving them: (a) for a coal miner; (b) for a child 10 years old.

COOKING AND PLANNING MEALS

Calculate the complete nutritional value of a cake by weighing the ingredients provided.
Weigh out amounts of (a) the baked cake and bread (b) boiled potatoes and chips to provide 300 kcal.
Weigh out amounts of boiled cabbage and salad both containing 30 mg of vitamin C.
With the ingredients provided, put together a meal containing 1,000 kcal, 25 g or more of protein, 200 mg or more of calcium, 250 µg of vitamin A and at least 10 mg of vitamin C.
Calculate how much food would be needed to supply 500 such meals.

Appendix D

RECOMMENDED BOOKS

W. R. AYKROYD. *Food for Man.* Pergamon Press. 1964. £0.45 (Paper), £0.75 (Clothbound).

M. E. BECK. *Nutrition and Dietetics for Nurses.* 3rd revised Ed. Churchill-Livingstone 1971. £1.00

A. E. BENDER. *Dictionary of Nutrition and Food Technology.* 3rd Ed. Butterworth 1968. £3.00.

A. M. BROWN. *Practical Nutrition for Nurses.* Heinemann Medical Books 1966. £0.75.

SIR S. DAVIDSON, R. PASSMORE and J. F. BROCK. *Human Nutrition and Dietetics.* Churchill Livingstone 1972. £6.00.

J. C. DRUMMOND and ANNE WILBRAHAM. *The Englishman's Food.* A history of five centuries of English diet, revised and with a new chapter by Dorothy Hollingsworth. Jonathan Cape 1958. £3.25.

J. V. G. A. DURNIN and R. PASSMORE. *Energy, Work and Leisure.* Heinemann Educational Books Ltd. 1967 £1.25.

B. A. FOX and A. G. CAMERON. *Food Science.* 2nd revised ed. of Chemical Approach to Food and Nutrition. University of London Press. 1970. £1.75.

HOWARD, A. N. and MCLEAN BAIRD I. (Eds.). *Nutritional Deficiences in Modern Society.* Newman Books 1973. £1.30.

MINISTRY OF TECHNOLOGY: NATIONAL PHYSICAL LABORATORY. *Changing to the Metric System: Conversion Factors, Symbols and Definitions.* 4th Ed. P. Anderton & P. H. Bigg. H.M.S.O. 1972. £0.40.

V. H. MOTTRAM. *Human Nutrition.* 3rd Ed. Edward Arnold. 1972. £1.75.

B. NILSON. *Cooking for Special Diets.* Penguin Books. 1972. 60p.

MAGNUS PYKE. *Food and Society.* John Murray. 1968. £1.50

MAGNUS PYKE *Food Science and Technology* John Murray 3rd revised Ed. 1970. £2.50.

MAGNUS PYKE. *Synthetic Food.* John Murray. 1970. £2.25.

H. M. SINCLAIR and D. F. HOLLINGSWORTH (eds.) *Hutchison's Food and the Principles of Nutrition.* 12th Ed. Edward Arnold. 1969 £6.75.

REPORTS

DEPARTMENT OF HEALTH AND SOCIAL SECURITY. Recommended Intakes of Nutrients for the United Kingdom. *Reports on Public Health & Medical Subjects No. 120.* H.M.S.O. 1969. £0.27½.

MINISTRY OF AGRICULTURE, FISHERIES AND FOOD. *Household Food Consumption and Expenditure 1972. Annual Report of the National Food Survey Committee.* H.M.S.O. 1974. £1.85.

NATIONAL RESEARCH COUNCIL. *Recommended Dietary Allowances;* a report of the Food and Nutrition Board. 7th revised Ed. National Academy of Sciences and National Research Council Publication No. 1694. National Academy of Sciences. 1968.

FOOD TABLES

R. A. MCCANCE and E. M. WIDDOWSON. *The Composition of Foods.* Medical Research Council Special Report Series No. 297. H.M.S.O. 1967. £2.40.

B. K. WATT and A. L. MERRILL. *Composition of Foods.* Agriculture Handbook No. 8. U.S. Department of Agriculture. 1963.

JOURNALS

Nutrition. Bi-monthly. Newman Books Ltd., 48 Poland St. W.1. £5.00 per year (Individual copies £1.00).

Proceedings of the Nutrition Society. 3 times a year. Cambridge University Press. £11.00 per year.

Nutrition and Food Science. Quarterly. Forbes Publications Ltd., Hartree House, Queensway, London, W.2. £1.20 per year.

Index

	Page
Absorption	21, 23, 34, 35, 37
Adrenaline	39
Amino acids	9
essential	10
Arachidonic acid	8
Ascorbic acid	31
Adolescent, diet	67
Adult diet	40, 65, 67
Alcohol	12, 50
Allergy, food	68
Aluminium	60
Amylase	37
Amylopectin	6
Amylose	6
Anaemia	22, 30
Appetite	35
'As purchased'	45, 62
Athletes, diets suitable for	67
B group vitamins	27
Bacon	13, 29, 52
Bacterial synthesis	31
Beriberi	28
Beverages	51
Bile	37
Biotin	31
Biscuits, effect of cooking	58
Blood sugar	39
Body-building foods	71
Bones and calcium	21
vitamin D	26
Books, recommended	102
Bran	22
Bread—source of carbohydrate	7, 45
white	28, 57
wholemeal	28
Bread and Flour Regulations	46
Butter	47, 52
Butyric acid	8
Cabbage—carotene in	25
vitamin C in	32
effect of cooking	59
Cakes, effect of cooking	57
Cholecalciferol	26
Calcium	20
absorption of	21
effect of cooking	60
recommended intake	42
Calorie, see kilocalorie	4
Carbohydrates	1, 5
Carotene	24
Cellulose	6
Cereals	45, 52, 56
breakfast	58
Cheese	47, 52, 56
Chickens, broiler	48
Children, recommended nutrient intake	42
young, diet for	65
Chlorine	19
Chorleywood bread process	57
Climate, effect on energy requirement	15
Cobalt	30
Cofactor	3
Collagen	54
Colon	37
Contamination, metallic	60
Conversion factors	3, 12
Cooking—effects of	53
losses	53
Cooking utensils, effect on food	60
Copper	24, 60
Cream	47
Creta praeparata	46
Cysteine	23
Dairy produce	47
Dehydrated vegetables	49
Dental caries	7, 21, 25, 65
Dextrin	6
Diabetes	39
Diet—adequacy (Table 6)	44, 68, 69
adolescent	40, 67
adult	40, 65, 67
athlete	67
balanced	1, 65
children	65
old people	67
Digestion	34
Digestive juices	35
Disaccharides	5
Disease, deficiency	28
Duodenum	34, 36
'Edible Portion'	45, 62
Education in nutrition	71
Eggs	47, 52, 55
Energy—	12
effect of age	15
effect of occupation	16
effect of recreation	16
needs of the body	16
value of foods	13
value of nutrients	12

	Page
Enzymes	2
Extractives, meat	54
Fat	1, 7
digestion of	38
recommended intake	41
Fatty acids	7
essential	8
polyunsaturated	8
saturated	7
unsaturated	7
Fish	48, 55
canned	55
fatty	55
frozen	55
Flour	46, 56
extraction rate	46
fortification	46
Fluorine	23
Folic acid	30
Food, Tables of composition	45, 75
Fructose	5
Fruit	50, 52, 59
dried	50
Galactose	5
Gastric juice	36
Gelatin	10
Glucose	5
liquid	5
Gluten	57
Glycerol	7
Glycogen	6
Goitre	23
Goitrogens	23
Haemoglobin	22
Hydrogenation	7
Ileum	34, 36
Insulin	39
Intakes of nutrients, recommended	40
International units	3, 24
Intestinal juice	36
Intestine, large—absorption	38
digestion	37
small—absorption	37
digestion	36
Iodine	3, 23
Iron	22
absorption	23
content of milk	47
recommended intake	42
Irradiation of food	54
Jejunum	36
Joule	3

	Page
Kidney	48
Kilocalorie, definition	4
recommended intake	40
Kilogram	3
Kilojoule	3
Lactation, nutrient intake	42, 43
Lactose	5
Linoleic acid	8
Linolenic acid	8
Lipase	37
Litre	3
Liver	48
Lymph	38
Lysine	10
Magnesium	19
Maillard reaction	11
Malnutrition	2
Maltose	5
Manganese	24
Margarine	8, 25, 52
Meal(s)	61
calculation of nutrients (Table 5)	64
definition	61
planning	65
school	66
Meat	48, 52, 53
canned	54
dehydrated	54
frozen	54
Megajoule	3
Metabolism, basal	14
Methionine	10
Metric system	3
Milk	47, 52, 55
dried	55
effect of sunlight	29, 33
heat treated and processed	55
skim	47
UHT	55
Minerals	19
Mineral oils	8
Monosaccharides	5
Muscle	48
Myoglobin	53
National Food Survey	51
Niacin	27
Nicotinic acid	29
equivalents	29
recommended intake	42
Nutrient content of the diet	50
Table	52
Nutrients in foods	75
Nuts	50

	Page
Obesity	17, 67
Oesophagus	34
Oils,	8
fish	8, 25
mineral	8
vegetable	8
Oleic acid	8
Oxalic acid	22
Palmitic acid	8
Pancreas	36
Pantothenic acid	31
Parathyroid gland	21
Pasteurization	55
Peas	49
Pectin	7
Pellagra	30
Pepsin	36
Phosphorus	23
Phytic acid	22
Potassium	20
Potatoes	52
powder	49
pre-peeled	59
vitamin C in	32, 58
Poultry	48
Pregnancy, nutrient intake	42, 43
Protective foods	1, 71
Protein	1, 9
absorption	37
quality	10
recommended intake	42
Pyridoxine	30
Recommended nutrient intakes Tables 1 & 2	42, 43
Retinol equivalents	24
recommended intake	42
Riboflavine	29
recommended intake	42
Rickets	26
Saccharin	6
Salads	59
Saliva	35
Salt	19
School meals	66
Scurvy	31
Secretin	36
S.I. Units	3
Sodium	19
Sorbitol	6
Soup	54
Starch	6
Starvation	18
Stearic acid	8
Stock	54
Stomach	37
Sucrose	5
Sugar	5
Sulphur	19
Teeth	7, 20, 23, 24
Thiamine	28, 52
recommended intake	42
Thyroid gland	19
Toast	57
Triglyceride	7
Trypsin	37
Tryptophan	10, 29
Urea	39
Vegetables—composition	49
canned	59
dehydrated	49
dried	49
effect of cooking	58
frozen	59
green	49
pre-peeled	59
root	49
Vitamins, fat soluble	24, 25, 26, 27
water soluble	27, 28, 29, 30, 31, 32, 33
Vitamin A	24
recommended intake	42
Vitamin B group	27
effect of cooking	28, 29
recommended intake	42
Vitamin B_{12}	30
Vitamin C	31
effect of cooking	31, 58
recommended intake	42
Vitamin D	26
recommended intake	42
Vitamin E	27
Vitamin K	27
Wastage of food	62
Water	2, 38
Weight control	17, 65
Wheat	45
germ	46
'strong'	56
'weak'	56
Yeast	57
Yoghurt	47
Zinc	24

Printed in England for Her Majesty's Stationery Office
by UDO (Litho) Ltd., London. Dd. 288610 K 240 2/75